EAT
YOURSELF
THIN

EAT YOURSELF THIN

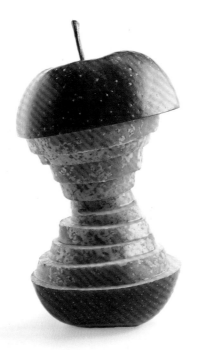

SUPERFOODS & RECIPES
TO BOOST METABOLISM & BURN FAT

GILL PAUL
NUTRITIONIST: KAREN SULLIVAN, ASET, VTCT, BSC

hamlyn

An Hachette UK Company
www.hachette.co.uk

First published in Great Britain in 2014 by Hamlyn,
a division of Octopus Publishing Group Ltd
Endeavour House
189 Shaftesbury Avenue
London WC2H 8JY
www.octopusbooks.co.uk

Gill Paul asserts the moral right to be identified as
the author of this work.

ISBN 978-0-60062-679-4

A CIP catalogue record for this book
is available from the British Library

Printed and bound in China

10 9 8 7 6 5 4 3 2 1

All reasonable care has been taken in the
preparation of this book but the information
it contains is not intended to take the place of
treatment by a qualified medical practitioner.

People with known nut allergies should avoid
recipes containing nuts or nut derivatives,
and vulnerable people should avoid dishes
containing raw or lightly cooked eggs.

Both metric and imperial measurements have been
given in all recipes. Use one set of measurements
only, and not a mixture of both.

Standard level spoon measurements
are used in all recipes
1 tablespoon = 15 ml spoon
1 teaspoon = 5 ml spoon

Ovens should be preheated to the specified
temperature – if using a fan-assisted oven,
follow the manufacturer's instructions for adjusting
the time and temperature. Large eggs should be
used unless otherwise stated.

Some of the recipes in this book have previously
appeared in other titles published by Hamlyn.

Art Director: Jonathan Christie
**Photographic Art Direction, Prop Styling
and Design:** Isabel de Cordova
Photography: Will Heap
Food Styling: Gee Charman
Editors: Katy Denny & Alex Stetter
Picture Library Manager: Jen Veall
Assistant Production Manager: Caroline Alberti

CONTENTS

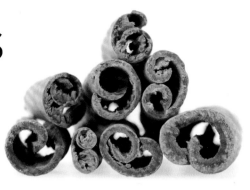

6   Introduction

PART I
10   **Thin superfoods**

12   **Superfoods**
Your key ingredients

26   **What's your problem?**
At-a-glance problem solver

30   **Putting it all together**
Weekly meal planner

PART II
34   **Thin recipes**

36   **Breakfast**
54   **Snacks**
68   **Lunch**
90   **Dinner**
110   **Desserts**

126   Resources
127   Index
128   Acknowledgements & Picture Credits

INTRODUCTION

It may seem a strange idea that you can eat yourself
thin, when eating made you overweight in the first
place. But it's not the process of eating that causes
weight gain, rather eating too much of the wrong
kinds of foods and drinking the wrong kinds of drinks.
This book shows you how to lose weight – and keep
it off – by focusing on foods that make your digestive,
hormonal and cardiovascular systems work at optimum
level, and on fluids that fully hydrate and replenish you.

Most weight-loss diets starve you. They tell
you to cut right back on calories, eliminate
carbs or skip meals – but all of these
approaches are almost certain to make
you regain the weight you've lost as soon
as you stop dieting. The body is designed
to maintain itself just the way it is – even if
it's overweight. If you cut back drastically
on your food intake, your body will
compensate by storing more of the calories
you do eat as fat. It's a mechanism designed
to save your life in times of famine, but it's
not so desirable when you've got three
months to shape up for a beach holiday.

How hormones affect weight

Hormones are the key to successful
long-term weight loss. Several different
hormones govern your appetite and
the way your body processes food.
....

● **Ghrelin and leptin** A hormone called
ghrelin tells the brain when you are hungry
and should eat more, while another
hormone called leptin tells the brain when

you are full. However, these hormones can
stop functioning properly in overweight
people, making them feel hungry even
after eating. To lose weight painlessly, it's
essential to get these hunger hormones
working effectively.
....

● **Insulin** Some foods are more likely to be
converted into fat in the body than others
because they cause blood sugar levels
to rise rapidly, making the body produce
insulin (see box, The Glycaemic Index).
Insulin is the hormone that converts food
into fuel for our muscles, and turns any
we don't need into fat to be stored for use
another day. High insulin levels make us
store more fuel as fat and make us continue
to feel hungry even when we've just eaten.
....

● **Cortisol** Another hormone that can
interfere with weight-loss efforts is cortisol.
High levels of cortisol, which is released
when we are stressed, cause increased
appetite and lead to more fat being laid
down around the waist, as well as making
us crave sugary, fatty foods for a quick

energy burst. But these sugary fatty foods only exacerbate the existing hormonal imbalances.

The way to break the pattern of cravings for unhealthy foods, or weight that piles back on again as soon as you stop dieting, is to get all your hormone levels back into balance. And to achieve that, the last thing you should do is 'shock' your body by starving it for a few weeks on a conventional diet. If you want to lose weight, and stay that way, you have to change the types of food you eat, and change them for good.

The Glycaemic Index and how to control cravings

The Glycaemic Index (GI) rates foods according to their effect on blood sugar. High-GI foods, such as sugar, alcohol and refined (white) flour products, are broken down quickly by the digestive system and cause blood sugar levels and insulin levels to soar, then plummet. Some people feel jittery and faint when levels drop, and get cravings to eat sugary, refined foods as soon as possible. The way to beat the cravings is to eat low-GI foods, such as wholegrains, pulses, fruits and vegetables, all of which will make you feel fuller for longer.

However, if you are a junk food or sugar addict, there is another reason to kick your habit, not just to lose weight. If you eat a lot of high-GI foods, the blood sugar/insulin mechanism can break down and cause insulin resistance, and eventually type-2 diabetes.

How to eat yourself thin

1. Eat regularly

Eat small, regular meals and snacks composed of low-GI foods (wholegrains, beans and lentils, vegetables) and high-quality protein (fish, eggs, poultry, lean meat, soya). These are digested slowly, meaning there is no spike in blood sugar levels and no excess insulin. This will also keep the leptin and ghrelin levels steady so you don't feel hungry. Try to eat something every three hours that you are awake. You'll have good energy levels, and the fibre in the low-GI foods will help to keep your digestive system working efficiently. Optimum digestion is one of the keys to sustained weight loss and overall health.

2. Avoid bad fats

Avoid unhealthy saturated fats (found in fatty and processed meats and bakery products containing palm oil) and trans-fats (found in spreads and many pre-packaged biscuits, cakes and pastries), but do eat foods containing healthy fats, such as olives, avocado, nuts, seeds and oily fish. Omega-3 fats found in fish such as salmon, herring, mackerel and sardines can help reduce hunger, as well as being good for your heart and circulatory system.

3. Choose soup for lunch

Soup is a nutritious appetite suppressant and an ideal lunch for those who are watching their weight. In studies at Penn State University in the US, it was found that ghrelin production was suppressed for at least twice as long in women who had a bowl of chicken and rice soup, than in those who ate a chicken and rice casserole.

4. Get some sleep

Good-quality sleep is very important for those who want to lose weight, because lack of sleep leads to the production of more ghrelin and less leptin, and also disrupts the glucose/insulin metabolism. Try to eat foods containing the amino acid tryptophan, such as chicken, cheese, eggs, oats and brown rice, to reduce stress and promote restful sleep.

5. Avoid processed foods

Cook from scratch as much as possible. Key nutrients are often removed from food when it is processed. Chromium, for example, is an important mineral for maintaining blood sugar and insulin levels, as well as keeping cholesterol at normal levels, but is often removed from foods in processing. Make sure you get enough from your diet by including onions, tomatoes, mushrooms and wholegrain cereals.

6. Look after your organs

The liver filters old hormones from the blood, but it's unable to do this efficiently if it is clogged up and overworked. That's just one of the reasons why drinking a lot of alcohol is not a good idea, whether trying to lose weight or not. Eat foods that support the liver (such as coconut, brown rice, wholegrains, root vegetables and apples) to support your weight-loss efforts, especially if your weight gain is due to menopause or pre-menstrual syndrome (PMS).

Iodine is crucial for the functioning of the thyroid gland which determines the metabolic rate. If your thyroid is even slightly underactive, you will gain weight easily and find it difficult to lose again. Good sources of iodine include seaweed, fish, eggs, onions and artichokes.

7. Stay hydrated

Drink plenty of still water during the day in order to stay hydrated. Herb teas are also good, and green tea can positively help weight loss. Cut right back on caffeine-containing drinks (such as coffee, black tea and colas) which stimulate the release of insulin.

Pure fruit juices can cause a blood sugar spike because of the fructose they contain, but adding some low-fat yogurt to make a smoothie brings down their GI rating. Avoid all sweetened and sports drinks – even water 'with a hint of fruit', which has a lot of artificial sweetener in it. And be aware that diet foods and drinks often contain high levels of sweeteners. Even though they are low in calories, the sweet taste seems to trick your brain into expecting sugar and cause it to release hormones accordingly.

8. Treat yourself

Include some treats in your diet. You don't want to feel as though you are living a life of denial. It helps if you choose treats that have some nutritional benefits, such as a couple of squares of dark chocolate, a fruity dessert or a small glass of red wine. Avoid junk foods, which are high in saturated fats, trans-fats and sugars without supplying any nutrition at all, and which also place a heavy load on the digestive system.

Getting started

You'll notice that there's no mention of calories, points or portion sizes in this book. You won't have to weigh precise quantities or sit poring over a calculator to work out whether you are allowed dessert. It's about developing a new relationship with food in which you avoid 'empty' calories and become aware of the effects on your body of each food or drink that passes your lips. You may even eat more than you have been doing in the past, because when you consume healthy foods, the body uses them up instead of laying them down as fat.

To start losing weight, follow the two-week programme on pages 30–33. This will teach you the basics and help you realize that it's not going to be so hard this time. If you have encountered specific problems when trying to lose weight in the past, check the problem solver on pages 26–29. It will tell you which foods to focus on, then you can read pages 12–25 for suggestions about ways you can include them in your diet. All of the foods listed in this book, and

used in the recipes, are designed to promote weight loss in some way, and incorporating them into your diet may be just what you need to kick-start the process.

To give yourself an even better chance of success, start following a regular exercise programme as well. Choose something you enjoy. Study after study has shown that dieters who exercise are much more likely to keep the weight off long term. You'll feel better as soon as you start following this healthy eating programme, combined with exercising most days. Looking after yourself boosts self-esteem, so you'll both look and feel great.

Keeping up the good work

At the end of the two-week programme, carry on eating in the same way: have three small meals and three small snacks a day, never letting more than three hours go by without having some nutritious low-GI food.

Don't keep hopping on the scales, because weight can fluctuate from day to day, but aim for a steady loss of not more than 0.5–1 kg (1–2 lb) per week. If you aren't beginning to lose weight after a month of eating healthily, you may need to reduce your portion sizes slightly, but don't make any sudden or drastic changes. Once you reach your target weight, carry on eating exactly as you have been, perhaps slightly increasing your portion sizes. And don't forget to have those treats! You'll find that your tastes will change once you get used to eating healthily and you won't crave heavy, fatty, sugary foods any more. When your body is working efficiently, maintaining a healthy weight comes naturally.

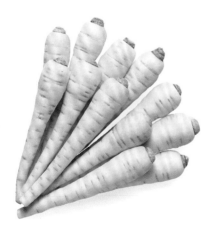

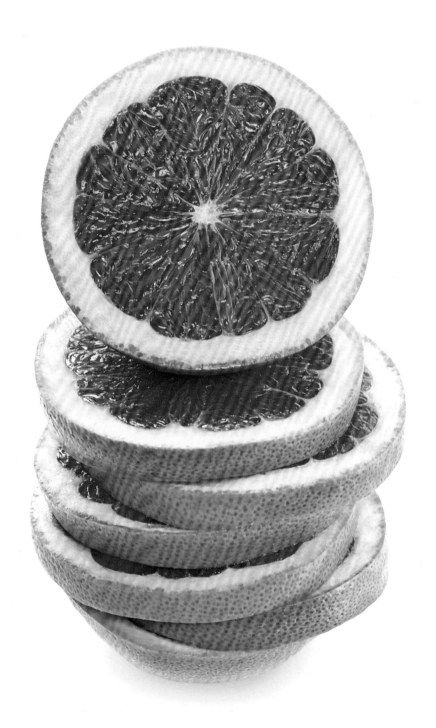

THIN
SUPERFOODS

SUPERFOODS

These are the key foods to focus on when you want to lose weight. Each one encourages the burning of fat cells and boosts the performance of every system in your body.

Blueberries

✔ Boost metabolism
✔ Reduce inflammation
✔ Lower cholesterol
✔ Balance blood sugar
✔ Prevent formation of new fat cells

Exciting research suggests that blueberries play a key role in preventing insulin resistance, which is implicated in diabetes and, in particular, belly fat formation. They also help to lower blood pressure and cholesterol.

They are rich in...
→ Fibre, to prevent constipation and improve nutrient uptake
→ Polyphenols, which prevent the development of fat cells
→ Anthocyanins, which reduce inflammation and improve health
→ Flavonoids, which boost the metabolism

Use in... breakfast juices and smoothies; bake into crumbles and stir into porridge; purée and serve with yogurt; add to wholegrain pancakes; toss into leafy green salads with a handful of toasted hazelnuts and some feta; use dried blueberries in place of raisins in salads, tagines and baked goods.

SEE: GREEN TEA PORRIDGE WITH BLUEBERRIES, P36; SUMMER BERRY GRANOLA, P38; CHICKEN & BLUEBERRY PASTA SALAD, P96; BLUEBERRY CHEESECAKE POTS, P114; CINNAMON BRIOCHE WITH MIXED BERRIES, P124.

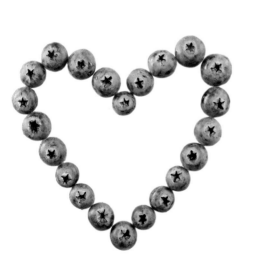

Green tea

✔ Promotes the loss of body fat
✔ Improves metabolism
✔ Encourages a sense of calm
✔ Reduces sugar cravings
✔ Supports liver function
✔ Lowers blood pressure

Green tea is rich in antioxidants which are known to help prevent several types of cancer and enhance metabolism. One study found that men who drank green tea daily had significantly smaller waist measurements, while another found that regular drinkers burn over 200 more calories per day than non-drinkers. It supports liver function, improving hormone balance, making it an excellent choice for anyone with hormone-related weight gain.

It's rich in...
→ Catechins, which encourage the loss of body fat and promote metabolism
→ Theanine, an amino acid which eases feelings of depression and lifts mood
→ Natural ACE inhibitors, to lower blood pressure
→ Antioxidants, which increase good cholesterol and lower high blood pressure

Use in... hot or cold drinks, with lemon, honey and/or mint; soak porridge oats or muesli in green tea instead of water or milk; blend with berries, honey and yogurt for a healthy smoothie; soak dried fruit in green tea and serve as a warm compote.

SEE: GREEN TEA PORRIDGE WITH BLUEBERRIES, P36; GREEN TEA & GINGER GRANITA, P120.

Cider vinegar

✔ Reduces appetite
✔ Encourages healthy digestion
✔ Stimulates metabolism
✔ Stabilizes blood sugar
✔ Prevents abdominal fat forming
✔ Reduces blood pressure

Apple cider vinegar is a natural digestive that can encourage healthy assimilation of food and also stimulate the metabolism. Several studies have found that it helps to lower blood sugar levels and blood pressure, and leaves you feeling more satisfied and fuller after a meal.

It's rich in...
→ Acetic acid, which suppresses appetite, prevents fat accumulation (particularly around the belly) and reduces blood pressure
→ Potassium, to improve brain and nervous system health, increase alertness and balance blood sugar levels
→ Pectin, which helps to regulate blood pressure and reduce bad cholesterol
→ Malic acid, which boosts energy levels and promotes liver function, thus balancing hormones

Use in... vinaigrettes with honey and olive oil; stir into a glass of hot water with honey; add to tomato sauces, soups and casseroles to lift flavour; use as a marinade for meat, fish and poultry; use to pickle beetroot for a nutrient-rich feast!

SEE: HUEVOS RANCHEROS, P50; CRANBERRY & APPLE SMOOTHIE, P64; CHILLED GAZPACHO, P74; LETTUCE WRAPPERS WITH CRAB, P82; CHICKEN BROCHETTES WITH CUCUMBER & KELP SALAD, P94; CHICKEN & APPLE STEW, P97.

Soya

✔ Promotes digestion
✔ Prevents constipation
✔ Balances hormones
✔ Reduces cholesterol
✔ Controls blood sugar levels
✔ Supports heart health

Soya (in the form of edamame beans, tofu, soya milk and soya yogurt) is an excellent source of protein, which will help you feel fuller for longer and provide a sustained source of energy. It also contains chemicals that have been shown to reduce the production of fat cells. It is one of only a few plant sources of omega-3 oils, which encourage overall health, and help to balance weight and mood.

It's rich in...

➜ Phytoestrogens, which can balance hormones, thus reducing hormonal bloating and weight gain
➜ Isoflavones, which reduce cholesterol levels and protect your heart
➜ Genistein, which reduces the size and production of fat cells
➜ Peptides, which improve blood pressure, control blood sugar levels and boost immune function

Use in... salads as steamed edamane beans with a zesty lime dressing; steam and toss edamame beans with olive oil, lemon and pepper; purée the beans as an alternative to hummus; stir-fry tofu with brightly coloured vegetables; serve soya milk or yogurt with porridge and fruit.

SEE: ROASTED EDAMAME BEANS, P56; BAKED TOFU STICKS, P58; VEGETABLE & TOFU STIR-FRY, P106.

Parsnips

✔ Balance blood sugar
✔ Encourage healthy digestion
✔ Lower cholesterol
✔ Ease constipation
✔ Reduce high blood pressure
✔ Support thyroid function

The high fibre content of parsnips, along with their sweet taste, helps to reduce hunger and keep you feeling fuller for longer. They are rich in B vitamins to support balanced moods and aid restful sleep and even ease the impact of stress.

They are rich in...

➜ Folic acid, for a healthy heart and nervous system and balanced moods
➜ Soluble fibre, which lowers cholesterol and helps to balance blood sugar levels
➜ Potassium, to regulate blood sugar and boost immunity
➜ Manganese, which is required for healthy thyroid function

Use in... stews, casseroles and soups with other root vegetables; purée as an accompaniment to fish, poultry and meat; roast with thyme and a drizzle of olive oil; mash as a topping for fish, chicken or vegetable pies.

SEE: SPLIT PEA & PARSNIP SOUP, P72; SPICY CARROT & LEMON SOUP, P76; SCALLOP, PARSNIP & CARROT SALAD, P84; CHEESY PORK WITH PARSNIP PURÉE, P102; MOROCCAN CHICKPEAS WITH CARROTS & DATES, P104.

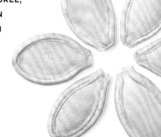

Rye

✔ Lifts mood
✔ Balances blood sugar
✔ Reduces fatigue
✔ Protects against heart disease
✔ Reduces appetite
✔ Lowers the risk of diabetes
✔ Prevents menopausal weight gain
✔ Promotes restful sleep

Rye is rich in fibre and studies have found that eating rye can reduce your daily calorie intake by up to 30 per cent. As a wholegrain, rye has a calming effect, boosting the production of feel-good hormone serotonin, promoting restful sleep and reducing symptoms of depression. It's a fantastic source of antioxidants too.

It's rich in...
→ Lignans, which promote heart health and improve digestion
→ Fibre, to reduce cholesterol levels, promote digestion, ease constipation and support healthy liver function
→ Magnesium, to support the nervous system and reduce the risk of diabetes
→ Chromium, to lower cholesterol and high blood sugar levels, reduce cravings, prevent type-2 diabetes and lower the risk of obesity

Use in... delicious sweet and savoury rye breads; toast rye bread as croûtons for hearty salads; bake in traditional cakes with fruit and honey; use rye berries in salads instead of rice or couscous; serve rye bread or crackers with smoked salmon, egg, tuna or chicken; use rye berries with herbs and feta to stuff roasted peppers.

SEE: POACHED EGGS & SPINACH, P48; TUNA PÂTÉ, P61; SWEDISH RYE COOKIES, P66; PUMPKIN SOUP, P73.

Pumpkin seeds

✔ Stabilize blood sugar levels
✔ Lift mood
✔ Increase energy
✔ Boost metabolism
✔ Promote restful sleep
✔ Encourage healthy thyroid function
✔ Reduce body fat

Pumpkin seeds contain minerals and amino acids which aid relaxation and sleep. This is helpful firstly because abdominal fat is exacerbated by stress. Secondly, those who lack good quality or adequate sleep are more likely to gain weight, partly because the hormones leptin and ghrelin are affected and these influence appetite.

They are rich in...
→ Magnesium, to support the nervous system and promote restful sleep
→ Tryptophan, which converts to serotonin to lift mood, relax and encourage sleep
→ Zinc, which stimulates the pituitary gland to produce thyroid-stimulating hormone (TSH) and boosts metabolism
→ Omega-3 oils, which help to decrease body fat by stimulating the enzymes that transport fat to the parts of the body where it can be burnt to produce energy

Use in... salads with ricotta cheese; sprinkle on cereals and porridge or use in muesli; lightly toast for a blood-sugar stabilizing snack; add to muffins or use to top homemade, wholegrain bread; add to fruit crumble toppings or sprinkle over vegetable gratins; stir into risottos.

SEE: SUMMER BERRY GRANOLA, P38; TURMERIC-ROASTED PUMPKIN SEEDS, P54; PUMPKIN SOUP, P73; PUMPKIN, FETA & PINE NUT SALAD, P86.

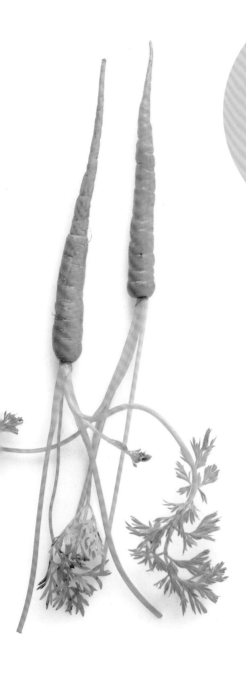

Carrots

- ✔ Reduce bloating
- ✔ Improve liver function
- ✔ Balance hormones
- ✔ Ease constipation
- ✔ Lower cholesterol
- ✔ Support heart health
- ✔ Boost immunity
- ✔ Enhance metabolism

Carrots stimulate and improve liver function, which is partly responsible for hormone balance in the body, as well as improving digestion and to some extent energy levels.

They are rich in...

→ Soluble fibre, which lowers blood cholesterol, balances blood sugar and promotes healthy digestion

→ Beta-carotene, to encourage the health of the heart and liver, boost immunity and speed metabolism

→ Sulphur, a key ingredient of insulin, which converts carbohydrates into energy and supports liver function

→ Vitamin K, for a healthy nervous system and brain function

Use in... stews, casseroles and soups; fruit and vegetable juices; roast with thyme and a little olive oil; serve raw with hummus for a satisfying snack; grate and drizzle with lemon vinaigrette for a tasty salad; grate and add to biscuits, muffins and cakes; stir-fry with fresh leafy greens.

SEE: SPICY CARROT & LEMON SOUP, P76; SCALLOP, PARSNIP & CARROT SALAD, P84; BAKED FISH WITH LEMON GRASS & GREEN PAPAYA SALAD, P93; LAMB & APRICOT TAGINE WITH PEARL BARLEY, P100; MOROCCAN CHICKPEAS WITH CARROTS & DATES, P104; VEGETABLE & TOFU STIR-FRY, P106.

Apples

✔ Reduce appetite
✔ Support liver function
✔ Boost immunity
✔ Balance blood sugar
✔ Ease constipation
✔ Promote digestion
✔ Provide long-term energy
✔ Support heart function

The carbohydrates in apples are digested slowly, helping to balance blood sugar levels and provide a feeling of fullness. One study found that overweight women who ate the equivalent of three small apples a day lost more weight on a low-calorie diet than women who didn't eat fruit.

They are rich in...

→ Antioxidants that can reduce the absorption of fat, and help prevent high blood pressure, insulin resistance (a precursor to diabetes) and obesity
→ Pectin, a soluble fibre which supports liver function and healthy digestion, and balances blood sugar
→ Quercetin, which reduces production of the stress hormone cortisol and supports brain and heart function
→ Polyphenols, which reduce the rate at which sugars are absorbed and stimulate the pancreas to release more insulin

Use in... stuffings for chicken, with seeds, nuts and wholemeal breadcrumbs; bake in crumbles with an oat, cinnamon and seed topping; add to fruit and vegetable juices; purée and serve with roasted meats.

SEE: APPLE, CINNAMON & ALMOND MUESLI, P40; CRANBERRY & APPLE SMOOTHIE, P64; CHICKEN & APPLE STEW, P97; ALMOND & APPLE CAKE WITH VANILLA YOGURT, P113; BAKED APPLES, P118.

Cinnamon

✔ Lowers blood sugar levels
✔ Reduces cravings
✔ Supports liver function
✔ Boosts metabolism
✔ Lowers cholesterol

Studies have found that just half a teaspoon of ground cinnamon a day balances blood sugar levels and reduces cravings. It also helps to reduce levels of the stress hormone cortisol, which can encourage belly fat and slow down metabolism.

It's rich in...

→ MCHP, which enhances the effects of insulin and so lowers blood sugar, reduces some forms of anxiety and lowers cholesterol
→ Sulphur, which supports the health of the liver and, through that, hormone balance, digestion and energy levels
→ Calcium, to encourage restful sleep and a healthy nervous system
→ Cinnamaldehyde, to balance hormones (in particular, testosterone and progesterone)

Use in... porridge; stir into freshly pressed apple juice; add to fruit purées and serve with live yogurt; add a teaspoon to chicken and lamb casseroles; steep cinnamon sticks in boiling water to make a stimulating tea; sprinkle over mashed bananas or puréed apples and serve on warm wholemeal toast.

SEE: APPLE, CINNAMON & ALMOND MUESLI, P40; CHICKEN & APPLE STEW, P97; LAMB & APRICOT TAGINE WITH PEARL BARLEY, P100; SLOW-COOKED SPICY BEEF, P103; MOROCCAN CHICKPEAS WITH CARROTS & DATES, P104; BAKED APPLES, P118; SLICED ORANGES WITH ALMONDS, P121; CINNAMON BRIOCHE WITH MIXED BERRIES, P124.

Almonds

✔ Promote fat burning
✔ Boost energy levels
✔ Balance blood sugar
✔ Lift mood
✔ Support the liver
✔ Prevent heart disease
✔ Promote relaxation
✔ Support thyroid function
✔ Aid restful sleep

High in fibre and protein, almonds provide a sustained source of energy and help to balance blood sugar levels, which is particularly helpful in dealing with belly fat. Research shows that people who regularly consume almonds have a healthier body weight than those who don't.

They are rich in...

→ Zinc and vitamin B12, to boost mood and stimulate the thyroid gland
→ Healthy fats, to fight heart disease and prevent insulin resistance
→ Calcium, magnesium and tryptophan, to encourage restful sleep and calm
→ Phytoestrogens, to balance hormones

Use in... salads with grapes and goats' cheese; spread almond butter on wholemeal crackers or toast; added to mueslis and granolas, or sprinkle over breakfast cereals; lightly toast and eat as a snack; chop and add to rice salads or as a crunchy topping for carrot or squash soup; use ground almonds in cakes and cookies.

APPLE, CINNAMON & ALMOND MUESLI, P40; BANANA & ALMOND SMOOTHIE, P46; CHICKEN & APPLE STEW, P97; MOROCCAN CHICKPEAS WITH CARROTS & DATES, P104; PUMPKIN CURRY WITH PINK GRAPEFRUIT SALAD, P107; ALMOND & APPLE CAKE WITH VANILLA YOGURT, P113; SLICED ORANGES WITH ALMONDS, P121.

Eggs

✔ Balance hormones
✔ Support the liver
✔ Boost energy levels
✔ Regulate appetite
✔ Balance blood sugar
✔ Reduce cravings
✔ Encourage thyroid health
✔ Lift mood
✔ Encourage restful sleep

The protein found in eggs contains all eight amino acids necessary for general health and, in particular, the ability to break down food for energy and regeneration. They also contain plenty of B vitamins, which help to control sugar cravings. Eating eggs for breakfast can reduce daily calorie intake by more than 400 calories. What's more, they contain iodine to support the thyroid gland.

They are rich in...

→ Choline, a soluble mineral which helps prevent fat from being laid down in the liver, thus improving hormone balance
→ Protein, to keep you fuller for longer, raise energy and balance sugar levels
→ Vitamin B12, to help metabolize fat
→ Folic acid, to lift mood and support the nervous system

Use in... salads and sandwich fillings; frittatas with peppers and goats' cheese; poach and serve on a bed of wilted spinach; soft-boil and serve with asparagus spears for dipping; use in cakes and baked goods.

SEE: LIGHT CRÊPES, P41; DATE & BANANA PANCAKES, P42; POACHED EGGS & SPINACH, P48; HUEVOS RANCHEROS, P50; MOROCCAN BAKED EGGS, P52; ASPARAGUS WITH SMOKED SALMON, P53; CHILLED GAZPACHO, P74; GREEN BEAN & ASPARAGUS SALAD, P85, SMOKED HADDOCK WITH POACHED EGGS, P92.

Lentils

✔ Reduce PMS bloating and cravings
✔ Stop abdominal fat being laid down
✔ Balance hormones
✔ Provide sustained energy
✔ Encourage calm
✔ Balance blood sugar
✔ Lift mood
✔ Encourage restful sleep

Rich in protein, lentils help to stabilize blood sugar levels and, through that, reduce belly fat by preventing spikes of insulin that cause your body to lay down excess fat. As natural phytoestrogens, they help to balance hormones and address hormone-related weight gain.

They are rich in...

→ Soluble fibre, to help stabilize blood sugar levels, while providing a steady source of energy

→ Magnesium, which decreases the release of the stress hormone cortisol
→ Protein, to provide sustained energy levels, promote a feeling of fullness, and balance blood sugar levels
→ Vitamins B1 and B2, to ease symptoms of PMS, including bloating, cravings and mood swings that may lead to comfort eating

Use in... soups, casseroles, tagines and curries; sauté ready-cooked lentils with walnut oil and a little sherry and top with grilled goats' cheese; heat and serve cooked lentils with lemon, olive oil and chives; use in fragrant dahls with paneer cheese; use as a bed for pan-fried scallops.

SEE: BUTTERNUT SQUASH, ROSEMARY & LENTIL SOUP, P77; THAI RED VEGETABLE CURRY WITH COCONUT RICE, P108.

Seaweeds

✔ Promote thyroid health
✔ Support the adrenal glands
✔ Balance hormones
✔ Boost energy
✔ Improve metabolism
✔ Reduce risk of heart disease
✔ Regulate blood sugar

All seaweeds, including kelp (kombu and wakame), nori, dulse, arame and Irish moss, are enormously nutrient-dense sea vegetables with a host of health benefits. With over 70 minerals and trace elements, and a number of amino acids, they encourage health and wellbeing. Perhaps most important is their role in supporting glands, such as the thyroid and pituitary, which play an important role in balancing hormones and, through that, metabolism.

They are rich in...

➔ Iodine, to regulate thyroid function and female hormones and encourage healthy metabolism
➔ Iron, to boost energy levels and ease fatigue
➔ Phytoestrogens, to balance hormones and address hormone-related weight gain
➔ Fibre and protein (including 21 amino acids), to balance blood sugar and support health on all levels

Use in... sushi; add to quiches or scrambled eggs; sprinkle dried flakes over food instead of salt; add kelp flakes to stews, casseroles and soups for extra flavour, nutrients and texture; eat kelp noodles with a light, lemony sauce.

SEE: ROASTED SEAWEED & SESAME SNACK, P57; CHICKEN BROCHETTES WITH CUCUMBER & KELP SALAD, P94.

Grapefruit

✔ Boosts metabolism
✔ Balances blood sugar
✔ Supports the liver
✔ Improves digestion
✔ Reduces fat stores
✔ Lowers cholesterol
✔ Eases constipation
✔ Raises energy levels
✔ Lifts mood

Grapefruit is a fibre-rich food that uses up more calories in digestion than it provides, thus helping to reduce fat deposits. It encourages metabolism and helps you to feel full. One study found that people who ate half a grapefruit with every meal for 12 weeks lost an average of 1.5 kg (3 lb) in weight, while making no other changes to their diet.

It's rich in...

➔ Limonoids, which encourage the action of the liver, fight cancer and lower cholesterol
➔ Pectin, for healthy digestion and blood sugar levels, and lower cholesterol levels
➔ Lycopene (in pink and red grapefruit), to protect the heart and reduce the risk of diabetes
➔ Inositol, to promote the production and release of serotonin, and facilitate the metabolism of fats and cholesterol

Use in... salads with spinach and avocado; top with a little honey and cinnamon and pop under the grill; serve with fresh crab on a bed of rocket; purée a few segments with some mint leaves and crème fraîche for a delicious salad dressing.

SEE: GINGER-GRILLED GRAPEFRUIT WITH HONEY YOGURT, P44; PUMPKIN CURRY WITH PINK GRAPEFRUIT SALAD, P107.

Black beans

- ✔ Lift mood
- ✔ Encourage sleep
- ✔ Ease symptoms of PMS
- ✔ Raise energy levels
- ✔ Balance blood sugar
- ✔ Reduce appetite and cravings
- ✔ Support healthy digestion
- ✔ Ease constipation
- ✔ Lower cholesterol

→ Good-quality protein, to stabilize blood sugar levels, leave you feeling fuller for longer and provide energy
→ Soluble fibre, to encourage digestion, reduce the risk of heart disease and lower cholesterol
→ Anthocyanins, which lower blood pressure, protect the nervous system and digestive tract, encourage optimum brain function and balance blood sugar

Black beans are one of the most nutritious members of the pulse family. They are full of antioxidants, protein and fibre to support health on all levels and, in particular, encourage optimum digestion and prevent spikes of insulin that can lead to fat deposits.

Use in... burritos served in wholemeal tortillas with brown rice; use instead of meat or poultry in tacos; stir into soups, stews and casseroles; serve cold in a salad with sweetcorn, chopped peppers, avocados and a zesty lime dressing; use in spicy meat or vegetarian chilli.

They are rich in...
→ Magnesium, to boost serotonin levels in the brain and encourage restful sleep

SEE: BLACK BEAN HUMMUS, P60; BLACK BEAN SOUP, P70.

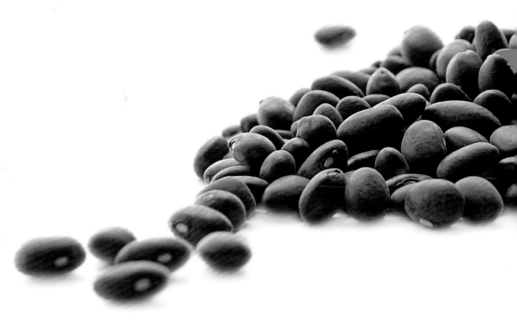

Tuna

✔ Improves heart health
✔ Lifts mood
✔ Supports the thyroid gland
✔ Lowers blood pressure
✔ Beats fatigue
✔ Reduces the impact of stress
✔ Balances blood sugar

Tuna has a host of health-giving properties, many of which address the factors that lead to obesity, such as comfort eating and low mood, poor-quality sleep, inadequate thyroid production and hormone-related problems such as PMS.

It's rich in...
→ Selenium, which supports thyroid function, lifts moods and encourages a healthy heart
→ Tyrosine, to raise energy levels, help deal with stress, produce thyroid hormones and balance mood
→ Omega-3 oils, to encourage heart and brain health, reduce symptoms of PMS and prevent surges in stress hormones that can lead to fat deposits
→ B vitamins, to produce serotonin, promote restful sleep and ease the symptoms of PMS and stress

Use in... a traditional salad niçoise; serve in a lemony sauce with wholemeal pasta; mix with chopped peppers, spring onions, chopped tomatoes and peas in a brown rice salad; mash tinned tuna with fat-free Greek yogurt and black beans and serve on toasted rye bread; grill fresh tuna steaks and serve on wholemeal buns.

SEE: TUNA PÂTÉ, P61; TUNA SKEWERS WITH COCONUT & MANGO SALAD, P90.

Turmeric

✔ Boosts metabolism
✔ Lowers blood sugar
✔ Encourages liver function
✔ Lowers cholesterol
✔ Breaks down fat
✔ Reduces the risk of diabetes
✔ Prevents bloating
✔ Improves digestion

By increasing bile production in the liver, turmeric boosts metabolism and lowers blood pressure, while breaking down fat deposits. It has also been shown to help prevent cancer, reduce bloating, improve digestion and lower cholesterol.

It's rich in...
→ Curcumin, which lowers cholesterol, boosts metabolism, promotes healthy liver function and breaks down fats
→ Sulphur, to support liver function and balance hormones, help prevent heart disease and improve digestion
→ Iron, to lift energy levels and banish fatigue that can be hampering weight-loss efforts
→ Manganese, for a healthy nervous system and energy production
→ Vitamin B6, which works with zinc to help metabolize food into energy

Use in... curries; add to soups and stews; use in piccalilli; add to omelettes; use in rice dishes and with pulses.

SEE: TURMERIC-ROASTED PUMPKIN SEEDS, P54; BLACK BEAN SOUP, P70; PUMPKIN SOUP, P73; TUNA SKEWERS WITH COCONUT & MANGO SALAD, P90; SLOW-COOKED SPICY BEEF, P103; MOROCCAN CHICKPEAS WITH CARROTS & DATES, P104; PUMPKIN CURRY WITH PINK GRAPEFRUIT SALAD, P107; THAI RED VEGETABLE CURRY WITH COCONUT RICE, P108.

Dates

✔ Reduce cholesterol
✔ Ease constipation
✔ Boost energy levels
✔ Improve digestion
✔ Lower blood pressure
✔ Balance blood sugar
✔ Boost metabolism
✔ Lift mood
✔ Support restful sleep

Dates have long been used to revitalize and supply energy – for example, when breaking the fast during the month of Ramadan. Rich in fibre, they help to optimize digestion and also prevent constipation. They are rich in tryptophan, to lift mood and encourage regenerative sleep.

They are rich in...

➔ Fibre, to reduce cholesterol levels, prevent constipation, balance blood sugar levels and ensure healthy digestion and absorption of nutrients
➔ Iron, to raise energy levels by improving the oxygen content of your blood
➔ Potassium, to lower blood pressure, regulate blood sugar levels and boost immunity
➔ B vitamins (in particular vitamin B6), which help the body metabolize carbohydrates, proteins and fats, ease symptoms of PMS (including bloating and cravings), promote a healthy nervous system and maintain healthy blood sugar levels

Use in... lamb and chicken tagines; flapjacks or biscuits; sticky toffee pudding; add to granola or muesli for breakfast; eat whole and fresh as a revitalizing snack.

SEE: DATE & BANANA PANCAKES, P42; MOROCCAN CHICKPEAS WITH CARROTS & DATES, P104.

Chicken

✔ Boosts metabolism
✔ Balances blood sugar
✔ Supports the thyroid gland
✔ Aids restful sleep
✔ Lifts mood
✔ Supports the liver

An excellent source of lean, good-quality protein, chicken is ideal for anyone wishing to lose weight. It boosts metabolism and prevents the storage of unwanted fat, while keeping you feeling full for longer.

It's rich in...

➔ B vitamins, which support energy metabolism and production, banishing fatigue and helping to balance mood, energy levels and blood sugar
➔ Selenium, which encourages the action of the thyroid, promotes a healthy immune system, lifts mood and protects your heart
➔ Phosphorus, which is necessary for the healthy functioning of the liver and nervous system
➔ Tryptophan, to encourage the release of the feel-good hormone serotonin and promote restful sleep

Use in... salads with plenty of crunchy vegetables; soups, casseroles, tagines and stews; stuff with apples, walnuts and wholemeal breadcrumbs and roast whole; stir-fry with Chinese vegetables and chillies; stuff chicken breasts with sun-dried tomatoes, ricotta cheese and spinach before baking; rub chicken portions with fragrant spices and serve with rice.

SEE: CHICKEN BROCHETTES WITH CUCUMBER & KELP SALAD, P94; CHICKEN & BLUEBERRY PASTA SALAD, P96; CHICKEN & APPLE STEW, P97; ROMAN CHICKEN WITH PEPPERS, P98.

Dark chocolate

✔ Balances blood sugar
✔ Lifts mood
✔ Reduces blood pressure
✔ Eases cravings and addictions
✔ Supports the nervous system
✔ Boosts energy levels
✔ Reduces stress

Dark chocolate is an amazing source of key nutrients, including iron, which boosts energy levels and helps to ensure a good supply of oxygen and nutrients to every cell in your body. Although the stearic acid in dark chocolate is a saturated fat, it does not raise cholesterol levels, but supports the nervous system and produces beneficial hormones.

It's rich in...
➜ Theobromine, which enhances physical and mental relaxation
➜ Anandamide, which raises levels of serotonin and feel-good chemicals known as endorphins
➜ Oleic acid, a cholesterol-busting fat
➜ Flavonoids, which help to reduce insulin resistance and stabilize blood sugar levels

Use in... sweet and savoury sauces and stews; choose chocolate bars with at least 70 per cent cocoa solids and grate on to fresh fruit or yogurt; snack on a handful of chocolate-covered brazil nuts; melt and blend with a banana and live yogurt for a rich, nutritious smoothie; dip fruit and nuts into a chocolate fondue for a satisfying dessert.

SEE: CHOCOLATE ESPRESSO POTS, P110; CHOCOLATE-DIPPED CHERRIES, P112.

Cheese

✔ Balances blood sugar
✔ Supports thyroid function
✔ Encourages restful sleep
✔ Lifts mood
✔ Aids relaxation
✔ Reduces cravings
✔ Provides relief from PMS
✔ Lowers blood pressure

Cheese is a satisfying, versatile food that is good for weight-loss programmes. It helps to reduce cravings for carbohydrates, and also lifts mood and promotes relaxing sleep. Opt for lower-fat cheeses such as mozzarella and Edam when possible.

It's rich in...
→ Tryptophan, which promotes the release of serotonin, helping you feel uplifted, while banishing cravings
→ Calcium, which lowers blood pressure, reduces symptoms of PMS and supports a healthy nervous system
→ Protein, to balance blood sugar levels, help you feel fuller for longer, raise energy levels and beat belly fat
→ B vitamins, in particular vitamin B12, which promote energy and the health of the nervous system

Use in... salads with apples, berries and crispy vegetables; stuff avocado halves with cottage cheese and top with toasted seeds; grate into a warming bowl of soup for extra nutrients; top vegetable bakes with grated cheese.

SEE: TUNA PÂTÉ, P61; SWEDISH RYE COOKIES, P66; PUMPKIN, FETA & PINE NUT SALAD, P86; RED PEPPER & FETA ROLLS WITH OLIVES, P88; CHICKEN & BLUEBERRY PASTA SALAD, P96; CHEESY PORK WITH PARSNIP PURÉE, P102; BLUEBERRY CHEESECAKE POTS, P114.

Coconut

✔ Regulates thyroid function
✔ Reduces cholesterol
✔ Eases constipation
✔ Raises energy levels
✔ Balances blood sugar
✔ Supports liver function
✔ Increases metabolism
✔ Reduces cravings

While coconut contains saturated fats, these have several health benefits and are easily metabolized by the body to provide long-term, sustainable energy. Coconut contains one of the few fats that can be heated to a high temperature without turning into an unhealthy trans-fat.

It's rich in...
→ Medium-chain triglycerides, a form of saturated fat that regulates thyroid function, improves blood sugar balance, promotes heart health and metabolizes quickly for sustainable energy
→ Fibre, to reduce cholesterol, encourage digestion and prevent constipation
→ Lauric acid, which boosts metabolism and supports immunity
→ Manganese, for a healthy nervous system, thyroid function and energy

Use in... curries and soups, in the form of coconut milk or grated fresh or desiccated coconut; use dried coconut flakes in muesli and granola; bake desiccated coconut into oaty flapjacks or wholemeal muffins; grate fresh coconut over sliced mango or serve in a salad with lime and ginger dressing.

SEE: PUMPKIN SOUP, P73; TUNA SKEWERS WITH COCONUT & MANGO SALAD, P90; PUMPKIN CURRY WITH PINK GRAPEFRUIT SALAD, P107; THAI RED VEGETABLE CURRY WITH COCONUT RICE, P108; COCONUT MANGO PUDDING, P116.

WHAT'S YOUR PROBLEM?

It may be that you have tried different diets in the past to no avail, or perhaps you have a health problem that contributes to excess weight. Decide which symptoms affect you and choose from the foods and recipes that can relieve them. There is an icon by each symptom. These icons are used in the recipes to highlight which recipes help combat which symptoms.

Fat around the middle

Blueberries, tuna, oranges, turkey, sweet potatoes, sunflower seeds, spinach, almonds, kale, eggs, broccoli, green tea, olives, avocado, lentils

Recipes Include: Green tea porridge with blueberries, p36; Scallop & broccoli broth, p68; Tuna skewers with coconut & mango salad, p90; Blueberry cheesecake pots, p114.

Menopausal weight gain

Salmon, tomatoes, barley, lentils, soya, spinach, oats, lentils, watermelon, quinoa, papaya, chickpeas, sardines, pumpkin, brown rice, walnuts, peaches, prunes

Recipes Include: Roasted edamame beans, p56; Raspberry, pineapple & papaya smoothie, p65; Butternut squash, rosemary & lentil soup, p77; Baked fish with lemon grass & green papaya salad, p93.

Post-pregnancy weight

Salmon, oats, blueberries, lentils, avocado, eggs, broccoli, almonds, oranges, quinoa, kidney beans, live yogurt, dark chocolate, chicken

Recipes Include: Summer berry granola, p38; Green bean & asparagus salad, p85; Chicken & apple stew, p97; Chocolate espresso pots, p110; Almond & apple cake with vanilla yogurt, p113.

Beer belly

Almonds, eggs, salmon, turkey, quinoa, oats, kale, flaxseeds, walnuts, seaweeds, soya, blueberries, raspberries, kiwi, sweet potatoes, dark chocolate, cheese, lentils

Recipes Include: Roasted edamame beans, p56; Chicken brochettes with cucumber & kelp salad, p94; Vegetable & tofu stir-fry, p106; Thai red vegetable curry, p108.

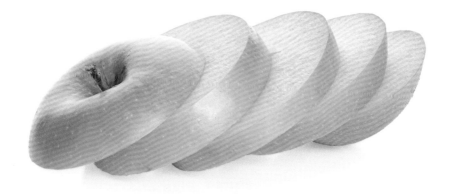

Cravings

Apricots, shellfish, peppermint, cheese, mackerel, pumpkin, chickpeas, eggs, dark chocolate, cod, broccoli, Romaine lettuce, cauliflower, tomatoes, chicory, cinnamon, apples, pinto beans, oats.
Recipes Include:
Apple, cinnamon & almond muesli, p40; Peppered beef with salad leaves, p78; Lamb & apricot tagine with pearl barley, p100; Moroccan chickpeas with carrots & dates, p104.

Fluctuating blood sugar

Almonds, quinoa, millet, avocado, walnuts, lentils, popcorn, peanuts, oats, apples, sweet potatoes, eggs, grapefruit, pumpkin, raspberries, apples, watermelon, dark chocolate, turmeric, sunflower seeds, cheese, cranberries, tomatoes, pumpkin seeds, lentils
Recipes Include:
Ginger-grilled grapefruit with honey yogurt, p44; Baked apples, p118.

High blood pressure

Celery, tomatoes, flaxseeds, bananas, spinach, mushrooms, butternut squash, seaweeds, papaya, live yogurt, kale, oats, eggs, soya, tuna, pork, garlic, peanuts, dates, parsnips, scallops
Recipes Include:
Poached eggs & spinach, p48; Scallop, parsnip & carrot salad, p84; Cheesy pork with parsnip purée, p102; Thai red vegetable curry with coconut rice, p108.

Stress

Asparagus, beef, milk, almonds, blueberries, tuna, dark chocolate, mango, mushrooms, beetroot, seaweeds, pumpkin seeds, brown rice, spinach, kiwi, chicken
Recipes Include:
Turmeric-roasted pumpkin seeds, p54; Peppered beef with salad leaves, p78; Green bean & asparagus salad, p85; Coconut mango pudding, p116.

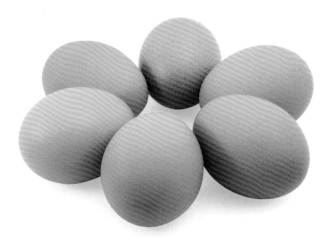

Low mood

Brazil nuts, spinach, oranges, grapefruit, herring, brown rice, spelt, soya, kidney beans, crab, turkey, green tea, apricots, almonds, lentils, blueberries, dark chocolate, sesame seeds, scallops, kale, pumpkin, aubergine, pumpkin seeds,
Recipes Include:
Ginger-grilled grapefruit with honey yogurt, p44; Aubergine dip with toasted tortillas, p62; Pumpkin curry with pink grapefruit salad, p107.

Underactive thyroid

Seaweeds, turkey, dark chocolate, prawns, beef, oysters, cashews, sunflower seeds, raspberries, eggs, tomatoes, coconut, red peppers, brazil nuts, live yogurt, chicken, oats, pumpkin seeds
Recipes Include:
Raspberry, pineapple & papaya smoothie, p65; Red pepper & feta rolls with olives, p88; Chicken brochettes with cucumber & kelp salad, p94.

Slow metabolism

Chillies, cherries, blueberries, milk, oats, quinoa, turkey, salmon, coffee, eggs, ginger, garlic, broccoli, almonds, grapefruit, pears, black beans, cider vinegar, turmeric, water, red meat, cinnamon, chicken, split peas, chickpeas
Recipes Include:
Turmeric-roasted pumpkin seeds, p54; Thai red vegetable curry, p108; Cinnamon brioche with mixed berries, p124.

Bloating

Live yogurt, tuna, asparagus, bananas, ginger, pineapple, papaya, green tea, peppermint, rye, fennel, watercress, melon, salmon, sunflower seeds, almonds, peppers, quinoa, cheese, turmeric, celery
Recipes Include:
Date & banana pancakes, p42; Banana & almond smoothie, p46; Baked fish with lemon grass & green papaya salad, p93; Green tea & ginger granita, p120.

Poor digestion

Live yogurt, black beans, pineapple, papaya, raspberries, artichokes, salmon, ginger, lentils, cider vinegar, peppers, brown rice, carrots, sweet potatoes, berries, oats, split peas, apples, rye, cranberries, dates, turmeric, parsnips
Recipes Include:
Raspberry, pineapple & papaya smoothie, p65; Black bean soup, p70; Thai red vegetable curry, p108.

Hormone imbalance

Flaxseeds, broccoli, kale, soya, quinoa, buckwheat, apples, coconut, oranges, turkey, walnuts, green tea, tomatoes, spinach, carrots, eggs, chickpeas, lentils, brown rice, rye, turmeric
Recipes Include:
Baked tofu sticks, p58; Spicy carrot & lemon soup, p76; Moroccan chickpeas with carrots & dates, p104; Vegetable & tofu stir-fry, p106; Green tea & ginger granita, p120.

Constant hunger

Chicken, soya, eggs, chickpeas, black beans, lentils, rye, whole wheat, dark chocolate, walnuts, almonds, peanuts, live yogurt, salmon, popcorn, coconut, cider vinegar, shellfish, pumpkin
Recipes Include:
Summer berry granola, p38; Huevos rancheros, p50; Asparagus with smoked salmon, p53; Black bean hummus, p60; Chocolate espresso pots, p110.

Low self-esteem

Blueberries, carrots, butternut squash, tomatoes, kale, spinach, Romaine lettuce, alfalfa, rye, cherries, grapes, tuna, salmon, dates, almond, chickpeas, lentils, broccoli
Recipes Include:
Date & banana pancakes, p42; Huevos rancheros, p50; Tuna pâté, p61; Moroccan chickpeas with carrots & dates, p104; Chocolate-dipped cherries, p112.

PUTTING IT ALL TOGETHER

Meal Planner	Monday	Tuesday	Wednesday
Breakfast	Fruity summer milkshake, p47	Summer berry granola, p38	Banana & almond smoothie, p46
Morning snack	Turmeric-roasted pumpkin seeds, p54	Cranberry & apple smoothie, p64	Swedish rye cookies, p66
Lunch	Scallop & broccoli broth, p68	Black bean soup, p70	Green bean & asparagus salad, p85
Afternoon snack	Aubergine dip with toasted tortillas, p62	Tuna pâté, p61	3 chocolate-covered brazil nuts
Dinner	Roman chicken with peppers, p98	Lamb & apricot tagine with pearl barley, p100	Chicken & blueberry pasta salad, p96
Dessert	Chocolate espresso pots, p110	Cinnamon brioche with mixed berries, p124	Green tea & ginger granita, p120

WEEK 1

Thursday	Friday	Saturday	Sunday
Asparagus with smoked salmon, p53	Green tea porridge with blueberries, p36	Light crêpes, p41	Poached eggs & spinach, p48
Chocolate-dipped cherries, p112	Black bean hummus, p60	Raspberry, pineapple & papaya smoothie, p65	5 dried apricots
Butternut squash, rosemary & lentil soup, p77	Scallop, parsnip & carrot salad, p84	Chilled gazpacho, p74	Pumpkin, feta & pine nut salad, p86
Baked tofu sticks, p58	1 hard-boiled egg	Roasted seaweed & sesame snack, p57	Roasted edamame beans, p56
Tuna skewers with coconut & mango salad, p90	Vegetable & tofu stir-fry, p106	Slow-cooked spicy beef, p103	Chicken brochettes with cucumber & kelp salad, p94
Almond & apple cake with vanilla yogurt, p113	Blueberry cheesecake pots, p114	Coconut mango pudding, p116	Sliced oranges with almonds, p121

Meal Planner	Monday	Tuesday	Wednesday
Breakfast	Apple, cinnamon & almond muesli, p40	Asparagus with smoked salmon, p53	Poached eggs & spinach, p48
Morning snack	1 hard-boiled egg	Turmeric-roasted pumpkin seeds, p54	Cottage cheese and sliced avocado on a rye crispbread
Lunch	Sushi rice salad, p80	Pumpkin soup, p73	Spicy carrot & lemon soup, p76
Afternoon snack	Aubergine dip with toasted tortillas, p62	Swedish rye cookies, p66	Cranberry & apple smoothie, p64
Dinner	Cheesy pork with parsnip purée, p62	Chicken & apple stew, p97	Thai red vegetable curry with coconut rice, p108
Dessert	Griddled peaches & apricots with honey yogurt, p122	Chocolate-dipped cherries, p112	Sliced oranges with almonds, p121

WEEK 2

	Thursday	Friday	Saturday	Sunday
	Ginger-grilled grapefruit with honey yogurt, p44	Huevos rancheros, p50	Date & banana pancakes, p42	Moroccan baked eggs, p52
	Baked tofu sticks, p58	Roasted edamame beans, p56	Raspberry, pineapple & papaya smoothie, p65	Black bean hummus, p60
	Lettuce wrappers with crab, p82	Split pea & parsnip soup, p72	Peppered beef with salad leaves, p78	Red pepper & feta rolls with olives, p88
	5 dried apricots	Tuna pâté, p61	Roasted seaweed & sesame snack, p57	3 chocolate-covered brazil nuts
	Smoked haddock with poached eggs, p92	Baked fish with lemon grass & green papaya salad, p93	Moroccan chickpeas with carrots & dates, p104	Pumpkin curry with pink grapefruit salad, p107
	Coconut mango pudding, p116	Baked apples, p116	Chocolate espresso pots, p110	Green tea & ginger granita, p120

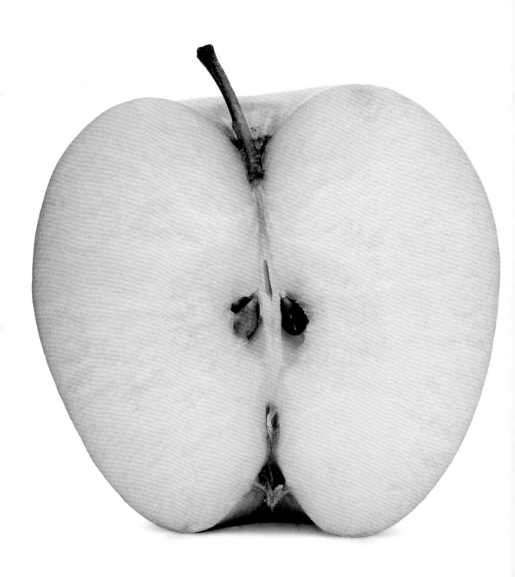

THIN
RECIPES

GREEN TEA PORRIDGE WITH BLUEBERRIES

An ingenious way to reap the health benefits of green tea, alongside fat-busting blueberries and deliciously soothing oats.

Preparation time: 5 minutes, plus steeping
Cooking time: 10 minutes
Serves 4
....

1.2 litres (2 pints) **water**
4 **green tea bags**
200 g (7 oz) **porridge oats**
100 g (3½ oz) **blueberries**
2 tbsps **low-fat live Greek yogurt**
2 tbsps **skimmed milk**
2 tbsps **maple syrup**

Place the measurement water in a large saucepan, bring to the boil and add the tea bags. Remove from the heat and allow to steep for 5 minutes.
....

Remove the tea bags and return to the heat. Stir in the porridge oats and return to the boil. Reduce the heat and simmer for 4–5 minutes, stirring frequently.
....

Add the blueberries and continue to cook for a further 2–3 minutes, or until the blueberries are warmed through and just starting to burst. Remove from the heat and divide between 4 serving bowls.
....

Thin the yogurt with the skimmed milk and pour over the porridge. Drizzle over the maple syrup and serve immediately.
....

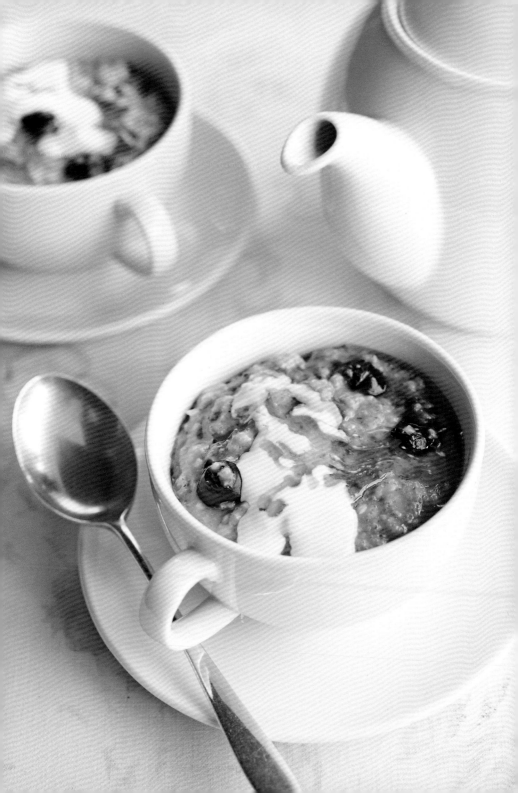

SUMMER BERRY GRANOLA

Serve this satisfying, energy-boosting granola with milk, yogurt and the berries of your choice.

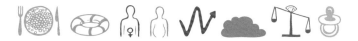

Preparation time: 10 minutes
Cooking time: 10 minutes
Serves 4
················

olive oil spray
200 g (7 oz) **porridge oats**
25 g (1 oz) **pumpkin seeds**
75 g (3 oz) **mixed nuts**, toasted
    and roughly chopped
1 tbsp **maple syrup**, plus extra to serve
300 ml (½ pint) **skimmed milk**
150 g (5 oz) **mixed summer berries**,
    including **blueberries** and **raspberries**
low-fat live Greek yogurt, to serve

Spray a baking sheet lightly with oil. Place the oats, seeds and nuts in a bowl and stir in the maple syrup. Spread the mixture out on the prepared baking sheet and place in a preheated oven, 180°C (350°F), Gas Mark 4, for 5 minutes.

················

Remove from the oven and stir well. Return to the oven and cook for a further 3–4 minutes until lightly toasted. Leave to cool.

················

Divide the granola between 4 serving bowls and pour over the milk. Top with the berries and serve with yogurt and a drizzle of maple syrup.

················

Any leftover granola can be stored in an airtight container for up to a week.

················

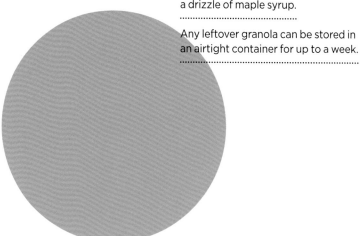

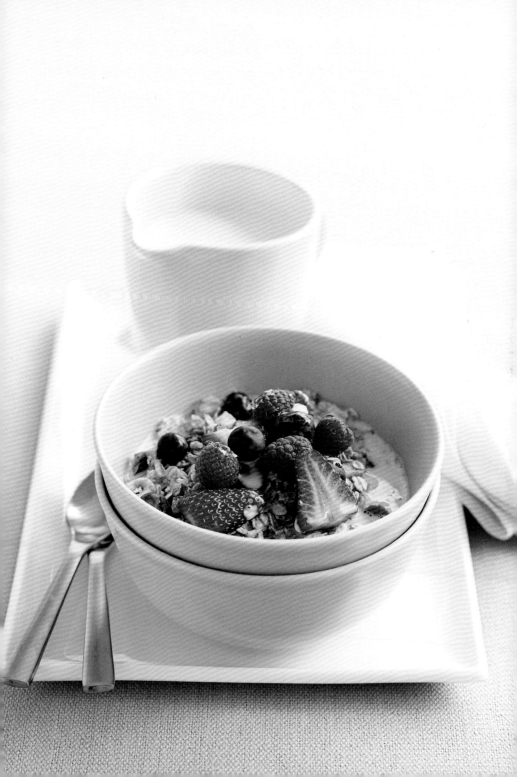

APPLE, CINNAMON & ALMOND MUESLI

Prepare this the evening before and refrigerate overnight for an instant energy-boosting breakfast, full of fat-busting nutrients.

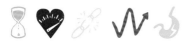

Preparation time: 10 minutes, plus chilling
Cooking time: 5 minutes (optional)
Serves 4
....

175 g (6 oz) **porridge oats**
250 ml (8 fl oz) **vanilla-flavoured soya milk**
250 ml (8 fl oz) **almond milk**
3 **red apples**, washed, cored and chopped
6 tbsps **almonds**, crushed
3 tbsps clear **honey**
1 tsp **ground cinnamon**

Place the oats and milks in a bowl, stir well and leave to stand for a few minutes. Stir in the apples, almonds, honey and cinnamon, cover and refrigerate overnight.

....

Serve cold, or warm gently in a saucepan or a microwave oven before serving.

....

LIGHT CRÊPES

These delicious crêpes can be topped with any fruit compote or fresh fruit. Sprinkle with cinnamon, sesame seeds or nuts.

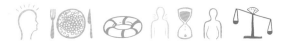

Preparation time: 10 minutes, plus standing
Cooking time: about 20 minutes
Serves 4
....

125 g (4 oz) **wholemeal flour**
1 **egg**
300 ml (½ pint) **skimmed milk**
1 tsp **vegetable oil**, plus extra for greasing

To serve
apple compote
ground cinnamon
cottage cheese

Sift the flour into a mixing bowl, then tip the bran in the sieve into the bowl. Beat the egg with the milk and oil, then slowly add to the flour, stirring constantly to form a smooth batter. Leave to stand for about 20 minutes, then stir again.
....

Heat a nonstick frying pan over a medium heat, then grease the pan with a little oil on a piece of kitchen paper. When the pan is hot, add 2 tbsps of the crêpe mixture and shake the pan so that it spreads.
....

Cook the crêpe for about 2 minutes until the underside is lightly browned, then flip or turn over and cook the other side for a minute or so.
....

Transfer to a plate and keep warm in a very low oven while you cook the remaining crêpes, stacking them one on top of the other as they are cooked. The mixture should make 8 crêpes in all.
....

Top the crêpes with apple compote, a sprinkling of cinnamon and a spoonful of cottage cheese, roll up and serve immediately.
....

DATE & BANANA PANCAKES

These fluffy American-style pancakes can be made the night before and reheated in the oven wrapped in foil.

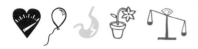

Preparation time: 15 minutes
Cooking time: 20 minutes
Serves 4

....

125 g (4 oz) **dried dates**,
    pitted and finely chopped
150 ml (¼ pint) boiling **water**
75 g (3 oz) **wholemeal** or **buckwheat flour**
75 g (3 oz) **plain flour**
1 tsp **baking powder**
½ tsp **salt**
1 tsp **ground cinnamon**
2 tbsps **golden caster sugar**
1 large **egg**
150 ml (¼ pint) **skimmed milk**
2 tbsps **olive oil**
2 tbsps **coconut oil**

To serve
2 ripe **bananas**, thinly sliced
maple syrup

Place the dates in a jug with the measurement boiling water and set aside to soak.

....

Meanwhile, place the flours in a mixing bowl with the baking powder, salt, cinnamon and sugar. Beat the egg with the milk and olive oil, then slowly add to the flour mixture, stirring constantly to form a smooth batter. Drain any excess liquid from the dates and stir into the pancake batter.

....

Heat a nonstick frying pan over medium heat and add a little coconut oil. When it starts to sizzle, pour in a little pancake batter. Cook for about 2 minutes until bubbles begin to appear on the surface, then carefully turn over with a spatula and cook the other side for a further minute.

....

Transfer to a plate and keep warm in a very low oven while you cook the remaining pancakes. Divide between warmed serving plates, top with sliced bananas and drizzle with maple syrup.

....

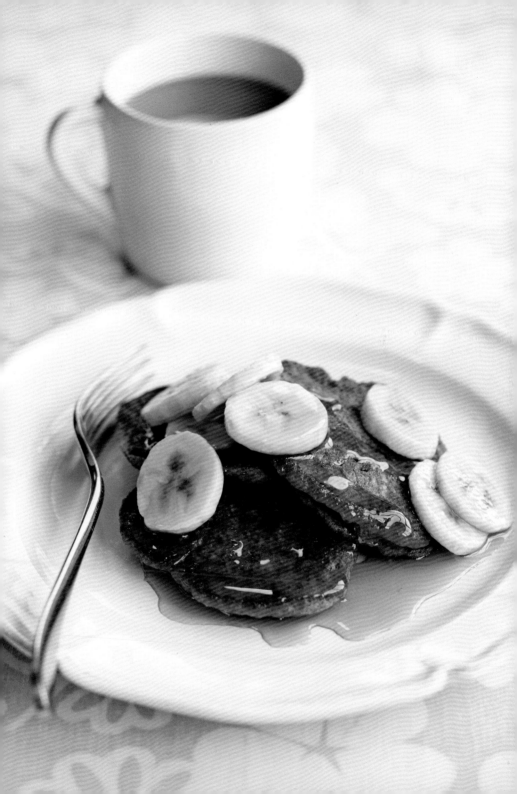

GINGER-GRILLED GRAPEFRUIT WITH HONEY YOGURT

A warming, healthy way to start the day, this fragrant grapefruit will kick-start the metabolism and lift the mood.

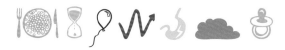

Preparation time: 5 minutes
Cooking time: 5 minutes
Serves 4
....

1 cm (½ inch) piece of **fresh root ginger**, peeled and finely grated
2 tbsps **brown sugar**
3 tbsps clear **honey**
2 **red** or **pink grapefruits**, halved horizontally
125 ml (4 fl oz) **low-fat live Greek yogurt**

Place the ginger and brown sugar in a small bowl, add 1 tsp of the honey and mix to a paste. Arrange the grapefruit halves on a grill pan, cut-side up, and spread with the ginger paste.
....

Place under a preheated hot grill for 5 minutes, or until lightly browned and bubbling. Meanwhile, mix together the yogurt and remaining honey.
....

Serve the hot grapefruit immediately, with the honeyed yogurt on the side.
....

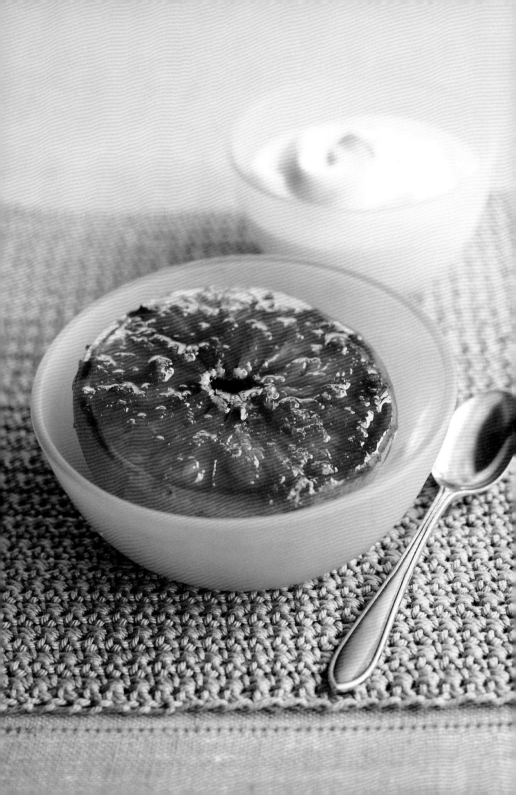

BANANA & ALMOND SMOOTHIE

Nourishing almond milk provides extra nutrients and protein in this filling smoothie, perfect for a sustaining breakfast.

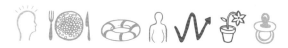

Preparation time: 5 minutes
Serves 4
....

325 ml (11 fl oz) **almond milk**
2 **bananas**, peeled and chopped
½ tsp **ground cinnamon**
½ tsp **vanilla extract**
6 **ice cubes**

Place all the ingredients in a blender or food processor and blend until smooth. Pour into tall glasses and serve immediately.
....

FRUITY SUMMER MILKSHAKE

This is the perfect breakfast for a busy morning, but also makes a good evening snack if you struggle to sleep.

Preparation time: 5 minutes
Serves 4
....

2 ripe **peaches**, halved, stoned and chopped
300 g (10 oz) **strawberries**
300 g (10 oz) **raspberries**
400 ml (14 fl oz) **skimmed milk**
ice cubes, to serve

Place the fruit in a blender or food processor and blend until smooth, scraping the mixture down from the sides of the bowl if necessary.
....

Add the milk and blend again until the mixture is smooth and frothy. Pour the milkshake over ice cubes in tall glasses and serve immediately.
....

POACHED EGGS & SPINACH

Eggs are an excellent way to start the day, ensuring you eat fewer calories and feel satisfied for longer.

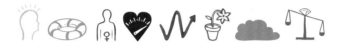

Preparation time: 5 minutes
Cooking time: 10 minutes
Serves 4
················

24 **cherry tomatoes** on the vine
2 tbsps **balsamic glaze**
small bunch of **basil**, leaves removed
4 large **eggs**
100 g (3½ oz) **baby leaf spinach**
sea salt and **black pepper**
4 thick slices of **rye bread**, toasted, to serve

Lay the cherry tomato vines in an ovenproof dish, drizzle with the balsamic glaze, scatter with the basil leaves and season to taste. Place in a preheated oven, 180°C (350°F), Gas Mark 4, for 8–10 minutes or until the tomatoes begin to collapse.

···

Meanwhile, bring a large saucepan of water to a gentle simmer. Carefully break 2 eggs into the water and cook for 3 minutes until the whites are just set. Remove with a slotted spoon and keep warm while cooking the remaining eggs.

···

Arrange the spinach on 4 serving plates and top each plate with a poached egg. Transfer the tomatoes to the plates and drizzle with any cooking juices. Serve immediately with the rye toast, cut into fingers.

···

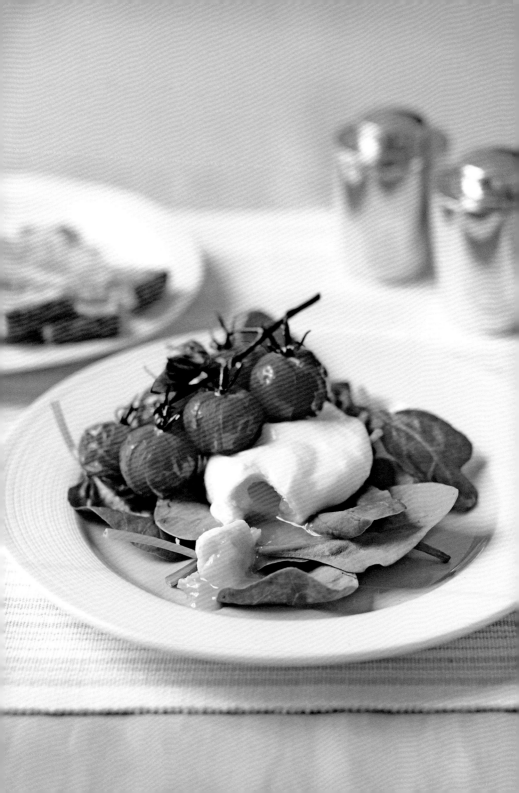

HUEVOS RANCHEROS

This twist on a Mexican classic takes just half an hour to cook and contains chromium-rich onions and tomatoes to balance blood sugar.

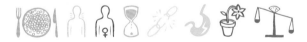

Preparation time: 15 minutes
Cooking time: 30 minutes
Serves 4
....

1 tbsp **olive oil**
2 **onions**, finely chopped
2 **red peppers**, cored, deseeded
    and finely chopped
4 **garlic cloves**, finely chopped
2 x 400 g (13 oz) cans **chopped tomatoes**
1 tsp chopped **oregano**
½ tsp **ground cumin**
1 **red chilli**, deseeded and finely chopped
1 tbsp **cider vinegar**
200 g (7 oz) can **black beans**,
    rinsed and drained
4 **eggs**
2 tbsps chopped fresh **coriander**
sea salt and **black pepper**
soft **wholemeal tortillas**, to serve

Heat the oil in a large saucepan over a medium heat, add the onions and cook for 5 minutes, or until softened. Add the peppers and garlic and cook for a further 5 minutes.

Stir in the tomatoes, oregano, cumin, chilli and vinegar and bring to the boil. Reduce the heat and simmer gently for 10 minutes.

Season to taste and stir in the beans. When the beans have warmed through, make 4 holes in the tomato mixture and crack an egg into each. Cover the pan and cook for 5 minutes, until the eggs have set.

Sprinkle with the coriander and serve immediately with warmed tortillas.

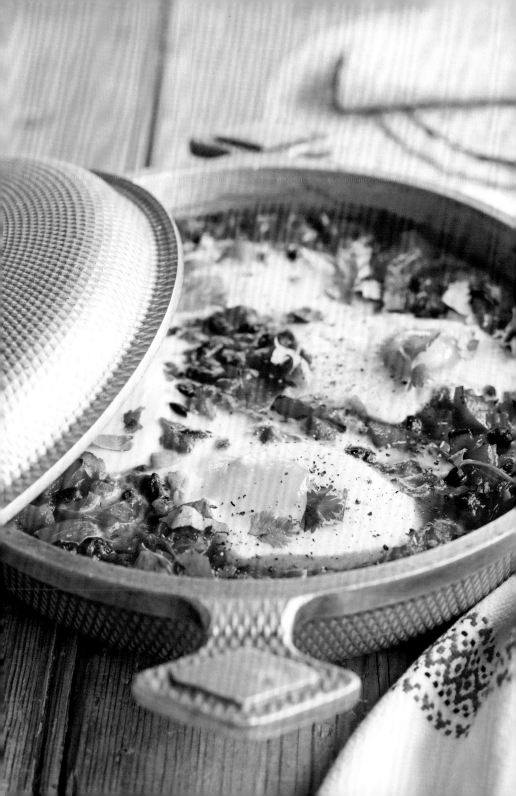

MOROCCAN BAKED EGGS

Perfect for brunch or a late, lazy breakfast, these gorgeous baked eggs will satisfy even the biggest appetite.

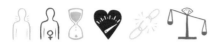

Preparation time: 10 minutes
Cooking time: 25–30 minutes
Serves 4

....

1 tbsp **olive oil**
1 **onion**, chopped
2 **garlic cloves**, sliced
1 tsp **ras el hanout spice mix**
¼ tsp **ground cinnamon**
1 tsp **ground coriander**
2 x 400 g (13 oz) cans **cherry tomatoes**
4 tbsps chopped fresh **coriander**
4 **eggs**
sea salt and **black pepper**
crusty bread, to serve

Heat the olive oil in a frying pan over a medium heat, add the onion and garlic and cook for 6–7 minutes or until softened and lightly golden, stirring occasionally.

....

Stir in the spices and cook for a further minute, then add the cherry tomatoes. Season generously and simmer gently for 8–10 minutes. Stir in 3 tbsps of the coriander.

....

Divide the tomato mixture between 4 individual ovenproof dishes, then crack an egg into each dish. Place in a preheated oven, 200°C (400°F), Gas Mark 6, for 8–10 minutes until the egg whites are just set. Cook for a further 2–3 minutes if you prefer the eggs to be cooked through.

....

Serve scattered with the remaining coriander and plenty of crusty bread on the side.

....

ASPARAGUS WITH SMOKED SALMON

This surprisingly low-calorie breakfast will help to reduce bloating, lift the mood and boost energy levels.

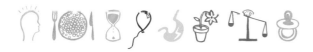

Preparation time: 10 minutes
Cooking time: 5–10 minutes
Serves 4
....

200 g (7 oz) **asparagus** spears, trimmed
3 tbsps roughly chopped **hazelnuts**
4 tsps **olive oil**
4 tbsps **lime juice**
1 tsp **Dijon mustard**
8 **quails' eggs**
200 g (7 oz) **smoked salmon**
sea salt and **black pepper**

Cook the asparagus spears in a steamer set over a saucepan of gently simmering water for 5 minutes until just tender.
....

Meanwhile, place the nuts on a foil-lined grill pan and place under a preheated medium grill until lightly browned. Place the oil, lime juice and mustard in a small bowl, season to taste and stir in the hot nuts. Set aside and keep warm.
....

Lower the eggs into a small saucepan of gently simmering water using a slotted spoon and cook for 1 minute. Remove from the heat and leave to stand for 1 minute, then drain the eggs, rinse in cold water and drain again.
....

Tear the salmon into strips and divide it between 4 serving plates, folding and twisting the strips attractively. Arrange the asparagus on the plates with the salmon.
....

Peel and halve the eggs and arrange on top of the salmon and asparagus. Drizzle with the warm nut dressing and serve sprinkled with a little black pepper.
....

TURMERIC-ROASTED PUMPKIN SEEDS

Great for thyroid function and attacking body fat, pumpkin seeds make an ideal snack at any time of day.

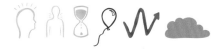

Preparation time: 10 minutes, plus cooling
Cooking time: 15–20 minutes
Serves 4
....

200 g (7 oz) **pumpkin seeds**
½ tsp **sea salt**
1 tsp **ground turmeric**
1 tsp **ground cumin**
1 tbsp **olive oil**

Place all the ingredients in a large bowl and toss until well coated, then spread out in an even layer on a baking sheet lined with baking paper.

....

Place in a preheated oven, 140°C (275°F), Gas Mark 1, for 15–20 minutes, or until the seeds are golden and beginning to pop. Allow to cool on the baking sheet before serving.
....

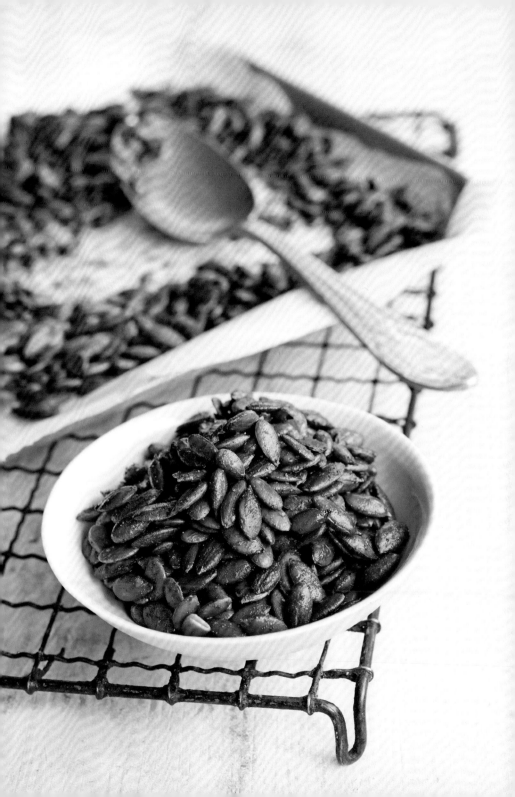

ROASTED EDAMAME BEANS

This is a great way to serve fibre-rich, hormone-balancing edamame beans (soya). Use fresh or frozen beans.

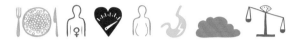

Preparation time: 10 minutes
Cooking time: 15 minutes
Serves 4
....

2 tsps **olive oil**
¼ tsp **dried basil**
½ tsp **chilli powder**
½ tsp **ground cumin**
¼ tsp **paprika**
½ tsp **black pepper**
250 g (8 oz) shelled **edamame beans**, defrosted if frozen

Place the oil, herbs and spices in a large bowl and use the back of a spoon to work into a smooth powder. Add the edamame beans and toss well to coat.

Spread out the beans on a baking sheet lined with baking paper and place in a preheated oven, 190°C (375°F), Gas Mark 5, for about 15 minutes, stirring once, until the beans begin to brown and smell fragrant.

Serve the beans warm or cold. Store any leftover beans in an airtight container.

ROASTED SEAWEED & SESAME SNACK

This is a good way to get thyroid-supporting seaweed into the diet. Use the sheets of nori seaweed that are used to wrap sushi.

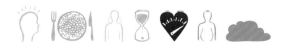

Preparation time: 10 minutes, plus marinating
Cooking time: 20 minutes
Serves 4–6

....

1 tbsp **olive oil**
1 tbsp **sesame oil**
1 tsp **lime juice**
½ tsp **sea salt**
8 sheets of **nori seaweed**

Place the olive oil, sesame oil, lime juice and salt in a small bowl and mix well. Lay a sheet of nori on a board and brush lightly with the oil mix.

....

Place a second sheet on top and repeat, then continue until all 8 sheets have been brushed with oil. Roll up the stack of nori and wrap tightly in clingfilm. Allow to marinate for 30–45 minutes.

....

Heat a nonstick frying pan over a medium heat. Place a sheet of nori in the pan and cook for about 1 minute, then turn over and cook the other side until the seaweed is crisp and toasted.

....

Transfer the toasted nori to a plate and repeat with the remaining sheets, stacking them one on top of the other on the plate as they are toasted.

....

Cut the stack into squares with a sharp knife, then separate the layers. Serve warm or cold.

....

BAKED TOFU STICKS

Serve these delicious snacks hot or cold to provide a hit of calming calcium and good-quality protein to keep you going through the day.

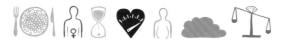

Preparation time: 10 minutes,
plus marinating
Cooking time: 30 minutes
Makes 24
....

400 g (13 oz) firm **tofu**
60 ml (2½ fl oz) **light soy sauce**,
plus extra to serve
150 ml (¼ pint) **water**
2.5 cm (1 inch) piece of fresh **root ginger**,
peeled and finely grated
3 **garlic cloves**, finely chopped
2 tbsps **sesame oil**
oil, for greasing
2 tbsps **sesame seeds**

Cut the tofu into 24 sticks and place in a shallow dish. Place the soy sauce, measurement water, ginger, garlic and sesame oil in a small bowl and whisk to combine. Pour over the tofu, covering it evenly, then leave to marinate for 30 minutes, turning once.

Transfer the sticks to a lightly greased baking sheet and sprinkle with the sesame seeds. Place in a preheated oven, 220°C (425°F), Gas Mark 7, for 15 minutes, basting with any remaining marinade if they look dry.

Turn the baking sheet and cook for a further 15 minutes, or until all of the liquid has been absorbed and the sticks are golden brown. Serve hot or cold with a little extra soy sauce for dipping.

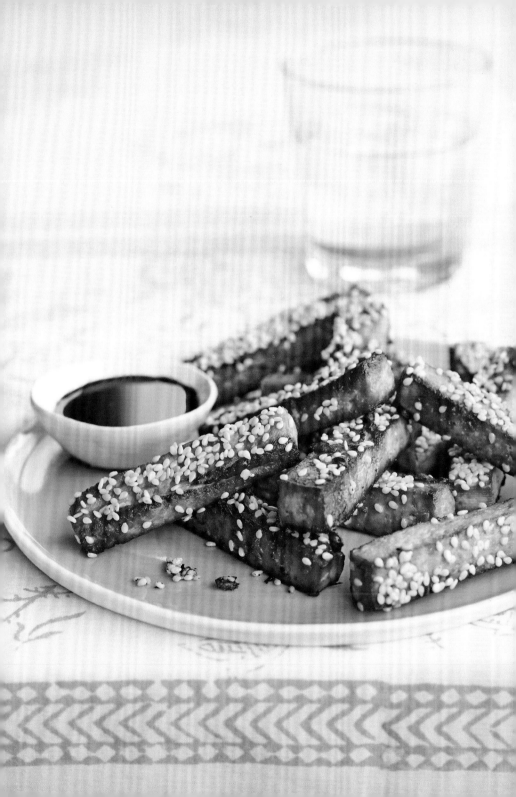

BLACK BEAN HUMMUS

This delicious hummus takes only minutes to prepare and provides a good boost of B vitamins.

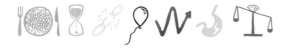

Preparation time: 5 minutes
Serves 4-6

....

400 g (13 oz) can **black beans**,
    rinsed and drained
finely grated rind and juice of 1 **lemon**
2 tbsps **tahini**
2 **garlic cloves**
1 tsp **ground cumin**
½ tsp **black pepper**
½ tsp **cayenne pepper**
½ tsp **paprika**, plus extra to garnish
12 **black olives** in brine, pitted,
    plus 2 tbsps of **brine**
carrot sticks, to serve

Place the beans in a blender or food processor, reserving a few for garnish. Add the remaining ingredients and blend until smooth.

....

Transfer to a serving bowl, top with the reserved beans and sprinkle with paprika. Serve with carrot sticks for dipping.

....

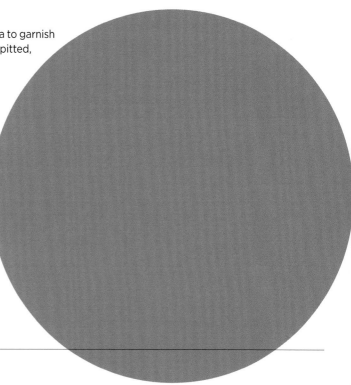

TUNA PÂTÉ

Rich in omega-3 oils to support heart health and beat fatigue, tuna makes the perfect pick-me-up snack.

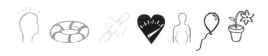

Preparation time: 10 minutes, plus chilling
Serves 4
················

200 g (7 oz) can **tuna** in spring water
100 g (3½ oz) **light cream cheese**
1 **spring onion**, finely chopped
finely grated rind and juice of 1 **lemon**
sea salt and **black pepper**
rye crackers, to serve

Place all the ingredients in a blender or food processor and pulse until almost smooth, but still with a little texture.
··

Transfer to a serving bowl and chill in the refrigerator for 20–30 minutes. Serve with rye crackers.
·······································

AUBERGINE DIP WITH TOASTED TORTILLAS

For extra flavour and nutrition, you could brush your tortillas with a little olive oil and sprinkle with sesame seeds before toasting.

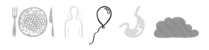

Preparation time: 15 minutes, plus cooling
Cooking time: 10–15 minutes
Serves 4

4 tbsps **olive oil**
1 tsp **ground cumin**
1 large **aubergine**, cut into 5 mm
    (¼ inch) thick slices
150 ml (¼ pint) **low-fat live Greek yogurt**
1 small **garlic clove**, crushed
2 tbsps chopped fresh **coriander**
1 tbsp **lemon juice**
4 soft **wholemeal tortillas**
sea salt and **black pepper**

Mix three-quarters of the oil with the cumin, season to taste and brush all over the aubergine slices. Cook in a preheated ridged griddle pan or under a preheated hot grill for 3–4 minutes on each side until charred and tender. Allow to cool.

Chop the aubergine finely and place in a bowl with the yogurt, garlic, coriander, lemon juice and remaining oil. Mix well, season to taste and transfer to a serving bowl.

Place the tortillas under a preheated hot grill for 1–2 minutes on each side until lightly toasted. Cut into triangles and serve immediately with the aubergine dip.

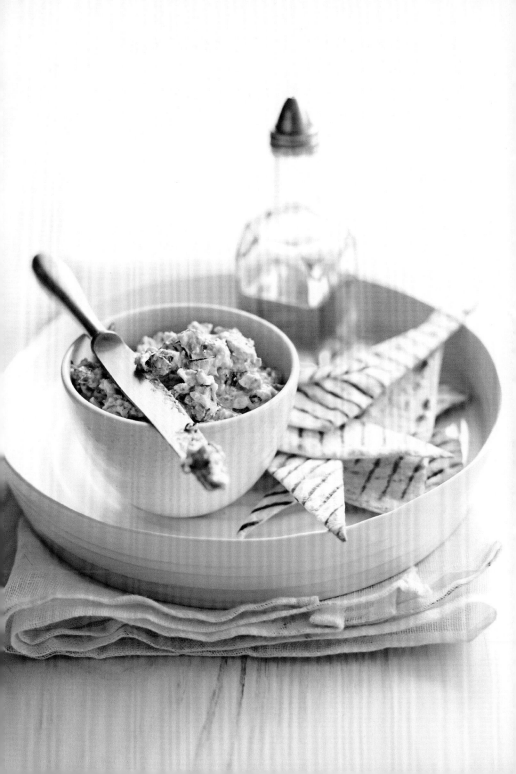

CRANBERRY & APPLE SMOOTHIE

Cranberries are all-round superfoods, boosting energy, balancing blood sugar, aiding digestion, promoting heart health and boosting immunity.

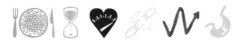

Preparation time: 10 minutes
Serves 4

1 kg (2 lb) **apples**
200 g (7 oz) frozen **cranberries**
1 tbsp **cider vinegar**
400 ml (14 fl oz) **low-fat live natural yogurt**
6 tbsps clear **honey**
ice cubes, to serve (optional)

Rinse the apples and chop them roughly, without removing the skin and cores. Juice the apple chunks in an electric juicer, or place in a blender or food processor and blend until smooth, then pass the juice through a fine sieve.

Transfer the apple juice to a blender or food processor, add the cranberries, vinegar, yogurt and honey and process briefly.

Pour the smoothie into tall glasses, add ice cubes, if using, and serve immediately.

RASPBERRY, PINEAPPLE & PAPAYA SMOOTHIE

This smoothie is guaranteed to nudge the digestive system and metabolism into action.

Preparation time: 10 minutes
Serves 4
....

1 **pineapple**, peeled and cut into chunks
1 large **papaya**, peeled, deseeded
    and cut into chunks
100 g (3½ oz) fresh or frozen **raspberries**
125 ml (4 fl oz) **orange juice**
1 tbsp chopped **mint**
10 **ice cubes** (optional)

Place all the ingredients, with the ice cubes, if using, in a blender or food processor and blend until smooth. Serve immediately in tall glasses.
....

SWEDISH RYE COOKIES

These crunchy cookies are rich in blood-sugar-balancing wholegrains and make an excellent snack or even a light dessert.

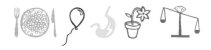

Preparation time: 20 minutes, plus chilling
Cooking time: 6–7 minutes
Makes 24
················

100 g (3½ oz) **rye flour**
100 g (3½ oz) **wholemeal flour**
½ tsp **sea salt**
100 g (3½ oz) **light cream cheese**
100 g (3½ oz) **unsalted butter**, softened
100 g (3½ oz) **golden caster sugar**,
   plus extra for dusting

Place the flours and salt in a mixing bowl, stir well to mix, then set aside. Place the cream cheese and butter in a separate bowl and beat with a hand-held electric mixer until fluffy.
····························

Add the sugar and continue beating until it has all been incorporated. Stir in the flour mixture until just combined.
······································

Turn out the dough on to a lightly floured surface and knead it briefly. Shape into a ball, wrap in clingfilm and chill in the refrigerator for 15 minutes until firm.
···································

Roll out the dough on a lightly floured surface to about 5 mm (¼ inch) thick. Use a 6 cm (2½ inch) cookie cutter or the top of a glass to cut out 24 rounds, rerolling the trimmings as required.
···································

Arrange the biscuits on 2 baking sheets lined with baking paper and place in a preheated oven, 180°C (350°F), Gas Mark 4, for 6–7 minutes until turning golden at the edges. Dust with caster sugar and allow to cool on the baking sheets.
···································

Store the cookies in an airtight container for up to a week.
····························

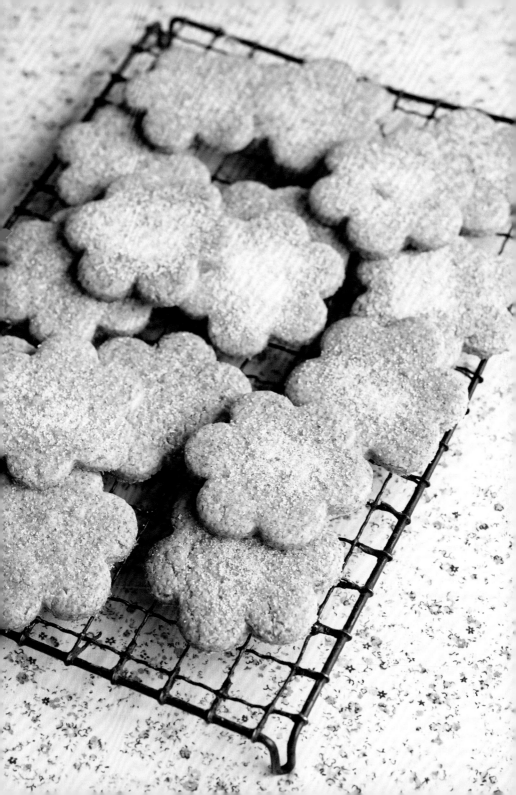

SCALLOP & BROCCOLI BROTH

Shellfish is a wonderful source of zinc, which helps to control appetite and encourage weight loss.

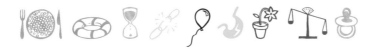

Preparation time: 10 minutes, plus steeping
Cooking time: 25 minutes
Serves 4

1.2 litres (2 pints) **vegetable** or
   chicken stock
25 g (1 oz) **fresh root ginger**, peeled
   and cut into matchsticks, peel reserved
1 tbsp **dark soy sauce**
3 **spring onions**, finely sliced
500 g (1 lb) **broccoli**, cut into small florets
1 small **red chilli**, deseeded and
   finely sliced (optional)
12 large **scallops** with roes
a few drops of **Thai fish sauce**
2 tbsps **lime juice**
sesame oil, to serve

Place the stock in a large saucepan over a high heat with the ginger peel and boil for 15 minutes. Set aside and allow to steep for a further 15 minutes.

Strain the stock into a clean saucepan, add the remaining ginger, the soy sauce, spring onions, broccoli and chilli, if using, and simmer for 5 minutes.

Add the scallops and simmer for a further 3 minutes or until just cooked through. Season with Thai fish sauce and lime juice and serve immediately with a few drops of sesame oil.

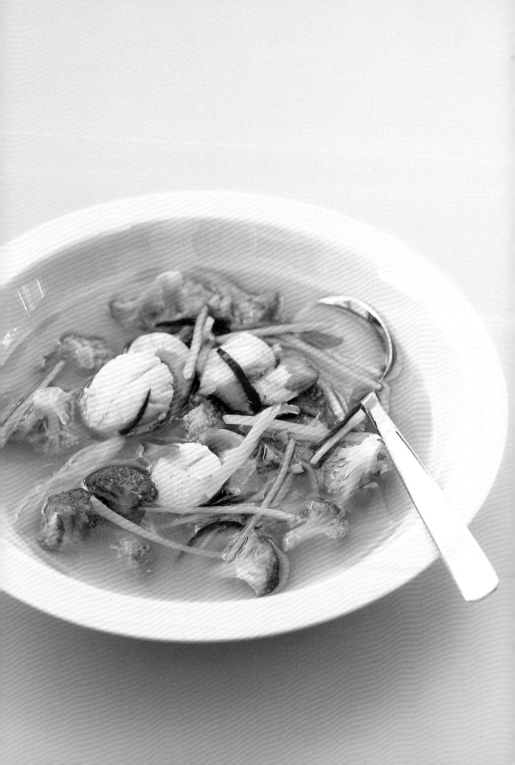

BLACK BEAN SOUP

Black beans are incredibly nutritious, providing a host of B vitamins, antioxidants and fibre to balance blood sugar.

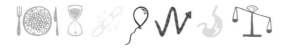

Preparation time: 15 minutes
Cooking time: 30 minutes
Serves 4
....

1 tbsp **olive oil**
1 large **onion**, chopped
2 tsps **cumin seeds**
2.5 cm (1 inch) piece of **fresh root ginger**, peeled and grated
4 **garlic cloves**, finely chopped
1 large **tomato**, chopped
2 tbsps **tomato purée**
2 tsps **ground turmeric**
600 ml (1 pint) **vegetable stock**
2 x 400 g (13 oz) cans **black beans**, rinsed and drained
sea salt and **black pepper**

To serve
handful of fresh **coriander**, chopped
4 tbsps **low-fat crème fraîche**

Heat the oil in a large saucepan over a medium heat, add the onion and cook for 5 minutes until softened. Add the cumin seeds, cook for a further 2–3 minutes.
....

Stir in the ginger, garlic and tomato and continue to cook, stirring frequently, until the tomato begins to break down. Add the tomato purée, turmeric, stock and half the beans and cook for a further 10 minutes.
....

Season to taste, place in a blender or food processor, in batches if necessary, and blend until smooth. Return to the pan, stir in the remaining beans and heat through. Transfer to warmed bowls and serve with a sprinkling of coriander and a swirl of crème fraîche.
....

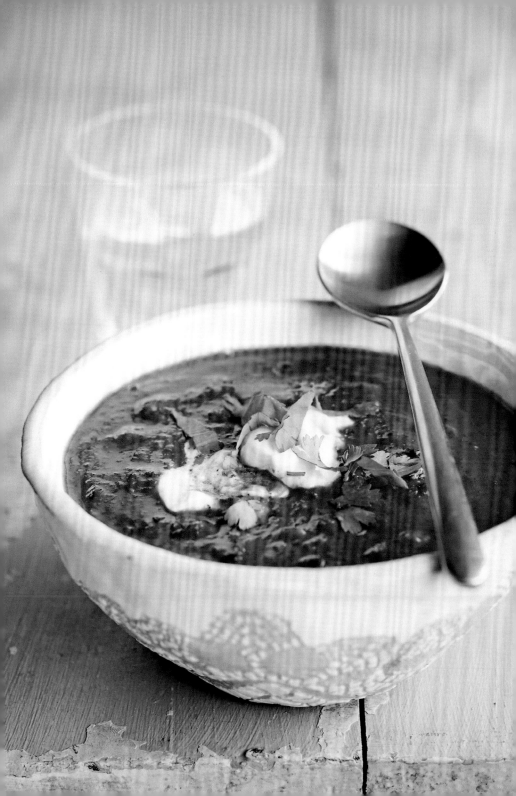

SPLIT PEA & PARSNIP SOUP

Chock-full of protein, fibre and B vitamins, this warming soup has a tasty knob of coriander butter on top as a treat.

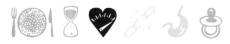

Preparation time: 20 minutes, plus soaking
Cooking time: 1¼ hours
Serves 4
....

200 g (7 oz) **yellow split peas**,
    soaked overnight in cold water
250 g (8 oz) unpeeled **parsnips**,
    cut into chunks
1 **onion**, roughly chopped
1.5 litres (2½ pints) **chicken**
    or **vegetable stock**
sea salt and **black pepper**
toasted **wholemeal pitta breads**, to serve

Coriander butter
1 tsp **cumin seeds**, roughly crushed
1 tsp **coriander seeds**, roughly crushed
1 **garlic clove**, finely chopped
50 g (2 oz) **butter**, softened
small bunch of fresh **coriander**,
    finely chopped

Drain the soaked split peas and place in a saucepan with the parsnips, onion and stock. Bring to the boil and cook for 10 minutes. Reduce the heat, cover and simmer for 1 hour or until the split peas are soft.

....

Meanwhile, make the coriander butter by dry-frying the cumin and coriander seeds and garlic in a small saucepan until lightly toasted. Mix into the butter with the chopped coriander and season to taste. Place on a piece of foil, shape into a sausage, wrap tightly and chill in the refrigerator until needed.

....

Roughly mash the soup with a potato masher, or place in batches in a blender or food processor and blend until smooth, if preferred. Reheat and stir in half the coriander butter until melted.

....

Add a little water if the soup is too thick, then season to taste. Ladle into warmed bowls and top each bowl with a slice of the coriander butter. Serve with toasted wholemeal pitta breads.

....

PUMPKIN SOUP

The slimming spices make this antioxidant-rich soup ideal for a weight-loss programme. Try it cold in the summer months.

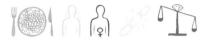

Preparation time: 20 minutes
Cooking time: 20 minutes
Serves 4
....

2 tbsps **olive oil**
1 tsp **cumin seeds**
1 tsp **ground turmeric**
1 tsp **ground coriander**
1 tsp **ground cinnamon**
2 small **red onions**, diced
2 **celery sticks**, chopped
2.5 cm (1 inch) piece of **fresh root ginger**,
	peeled and grated
1 **red chilli**, deseeded and finely sliced
3 **garlic cloves**, finely sliced
finely grated rind and juice of 2 **limes**
1 kg (2 lb) **pumpkin**, peeled,
	deseeded and diced
600 ml (1 pint) **vegetable stock**
400 ml (14 fl oz) can **low-fat coconut milk**
25 g (1 oz) fresh **coriander**, chopped,
	plus extra to serve
sea salt and **black pepper**

To serve
2 tbsps grated fresh or desiccated **coconut**
2 tbsps **pumpkin seeds**
toasted **rye bread**

Heat the olive oil in a large saucepan over a medium heat, add the cumin, turmeric, ground coriander and cinnamon and cook for 1 minute.
....

Add the onion, celery, ginger, chilli and garlic and cook for a further 4–5 minutes, then stir in the lime rind, pumpkin and stock. Bring to the boil, then reduce the heat, cover and simmer for about 8 minutes, or until the pumpkin is beginning to soften.
....

Stir in the coconut milk and continue to cook until the pumpkin starts to break up. Add the fresh coriander and the lime juice and remove from the heat.
....

Place the soup in a blender or food processor, in batches if necessary, and blend until smooth. Return to the pan, season to taste and heat through. Serve in warmed bowls, sprinkled with fresh coriander, grated coconut and pumpkin seeds, with toasted rye bread.
....

CHILLED GAZPACHO

This cold soup is surprisingly filling and the chopped egg will provide energy to see you through the afternoon.

Preparation time: 20 minutes, plus chilling
Serves 4

625 g (1¼ lb) ripe **tomatoes**
½ **cucumber**, roughly chopped
2 **red peppers**, cored, deseeded
    and roughly chopped
1 **celery stick**, chopped
2 **garlic cloves**, peeled
½ **red chilli**, deseeded and sliced
small handful of fresh **coriander**
    or **flat leaf parsley**, plus extra to serve
2 tbsps **cider vinegar**
2 tbsps **sun-dried tomato paste**
4 tbsps **olive oil**
sea salt

To serve
ice cubes
2 hard-boiled **eggs**, finely chopped
finely chopped **cucumber**,
    green pepper and **onion**
8 **blinis** (optional)

Place the tomatoes in a bowl and pour over boiling water to cover. Leave for 1–2 minutes, then drain, cut a cross at the stem end of each tomato, and peel off the skins.

Roughly chop the tomato flesh and mix with the cucumber, red peppers, celery, garlic, chilli and coriander or parsley. Stir in the vinegar, tomato paste and oil and season with salt.

Place the mixture in a blender or food processor, in batches if necessary, and blend until smooth. Taste and add more salt if necessary, then chill in the refrigerator for up to 24 hours until ready to serve.

Serve the soup in large bowls, scattered with ice cubes and chopped coriander or parsley. Place the chopped egg, cucumber, green pepper and onion in separate bowls and serve on the side with the blinis, if desired.

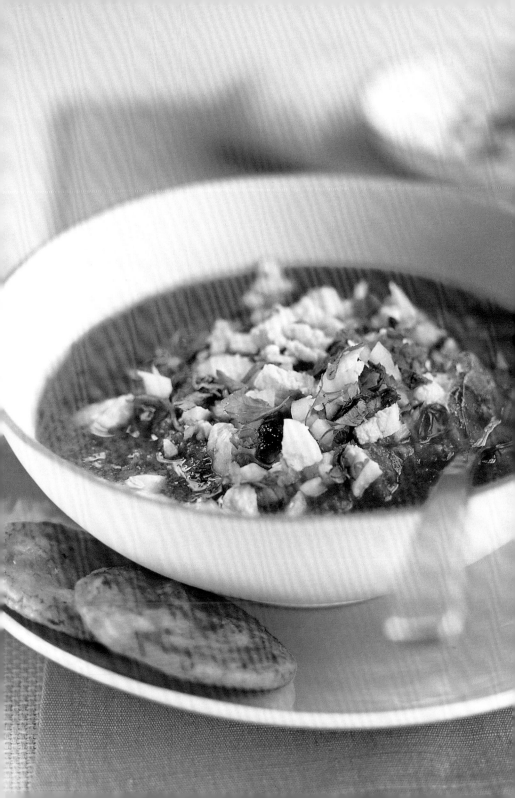

SPICY CARROT & LEMON SOUP

Warming, relaxing ginger, refreshing lemon and blood sugar balancing carrot come together in this delicious, satisfying soup.

Preparation time: 10 minutes
Cooking time: 30 minutes
Serves 4
....

2 tbsps **olive oil**
2 large **onions**, chopped
2.5 cm (1 inch) piece of **fresh root ginger**,
    peeled and finely grated
3 **garlic cloves**, finely chopped
625 g (1¼ lb) unpeeled **carrots**, sliced
2 unpeeled **parsnips**, sliced
finely grated rind and juice of 2 **lemons**
1.8 litres (3 pints) **vegetable stock**
sea salt and **black pepper**

To serve
2 tbsps chopped **parsley**
2 tbsps **low-fat crème fraîche** (optional)

Heat the olive oil in a large saucepan over a medium heat, add the onions and cook for 5 minutes until softened. Add the ginger and garlic and cook for a further 2 minutes.

....

Add the carrots, parsnips and lemon rind and continue to cook for another 1–2 minutes. Pour in the stock and bring to the boil, then reduce the heat and simmer for about 20 minutes until the carrots and parsnips are very tender.

....

Place the soup in a blender or food processor, in batches if necessary, and blend until smooth. Return to the pan, stir in the lemon juice and season to taste. Heat through.

....

Serve the soup in warmed bowls with a sprinkling of chopped parsley. Add a swirl of crème fraîche, if desired.

....

BUTTERNUT SQUASH, ROSEMARY & LENTIL SOUP

Antioxidant-rich butternut squash is complemented by hormone-balancing lentils in this flavoursome soup.

Preparation time: 10 minutes
Cooking time: 1¼ hours
Serves 4

....

1 **butternut squash**, peeled, deseeded and diced
a few **rosemary sprigs**, plus extra to garnish
2 tbsps **olive oil**
150 g (5 oz) **red lentils**, rinsed
1 **onion**, finely chopped
900 ml (1½ pints) **vegetable stock**
sea salt and **black pepper**
wholemeal rolls, to serve

Place the squash in a roasting tin with the rosemary, drizzle over the oil and season to taste. Place in a preheated oven, 200°C (400°F), Gas Mark 6, for 45 minutes until tender and golden.

....

Meanwhile, place the lentils in a saucepan and cover with water. Bring to the boil over a high heat and cook rapidly for 10 minutes. Drain, then return the lentils to a clean saucepan with the onion and stock and simmer for 5 minutes. Season to taste.

....

Mash the butternut squash with a fork and add to the soup, discarding the rosemary. Simmer for 25 minutes or until the lentils are tender. Ladle the soup into warmed bowls, garnish with rosemary sprigs and serve with wholemeal rolls.

....

PEPPERED BEEF WITH SALAD LEAVES

Beef is rich in iron to boost energy levels and fight fatigue, while mushrooms are rich in chromium to balance blood sugar.

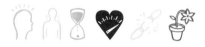

Preparation time: 15 minutes
Cooking time: about 5 minutes
Serves 4

500 g (1 lb) thick-cut **sirloin steak**
3 tsps **mixed peppercorns,**
   coarsely crushed
200 ml (7 fl oz) **low-fat live natural yogurt**
1–1½ tsps **horseradish sauce**
1 **garlic clove**, crushed
150 g (5 oz) **mixed salad leaves,**
   including Romaine lettuce
100 g (3½ oz) **button mushrooms**, sliced
1 **red onion**, thinly sliced
1 tbsp **olive oil**
sea salt and **black pepper**

Trim the fat from the steak and rub the meat with the crushed peppercorns and some sea salt.

Mix the yogurt with the horseradish sauce and garlic and season to taste. Toss gently with the salad leaves, mushrooms and most of the red onion and divide between 4 serving plates.

Heat the oil in a frying pan over a high heat, add the steak and cook for 2 minutes until browned underneath. Turn over and cook for a further 2 minutes for medium-rare steak, 3–4 minutes for medium or 5 minutes for well done.

Slice the meat thinly and arrange the slices on top of the salads. Serve immediately, garnished with the remaining red onion.

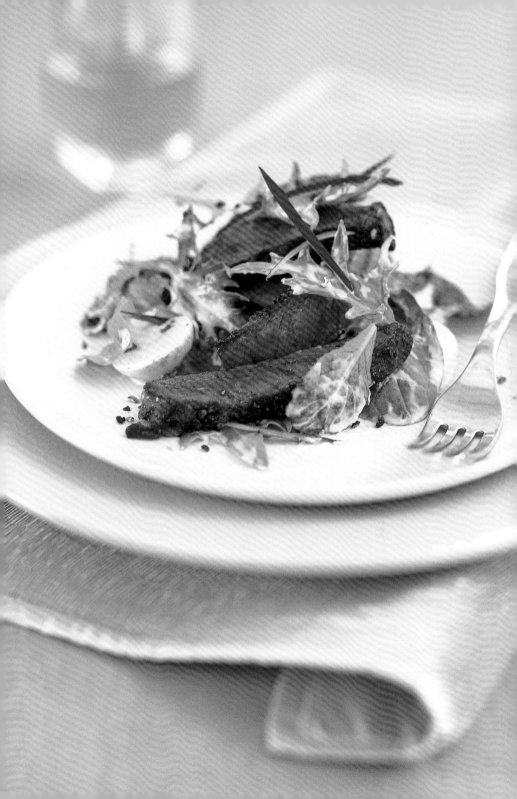

SUSHI RICE SALAD

This tasty salad is rich in nutrients that support weight loss, lift mood and aid relaxation. Use seared tuna instead of raw salmon if you prefer.

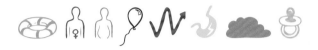

Preparation time: 20 minutes, plus cooling
Cooking time: 30 minutes
Serves 4

6 tbsps **rice wine vinegar**
2½ tbsps **caster sugar**
5 g (¼ oz) **Japanese pickled ginger**, finely chopped
½ tsp **wasabi paste**
½ **cucumber**
250 g (8 oz) **sushi rice**
250 g (8 oz) skinless, boneless **salmon**, cut into bite-size pieces
2 **avocados**, peeled, stoned and cubed
8 **spring onions**, finely sliced
4 tbsps **toasted sesame seeds**

Place the vinegar and sugar in a small saucepan and heat gently, stirring, until the sugar has dissolved. Remove from the heat and add the pickled ginger and wasabi. Leave to cool.

Cut the cucumber in half lengthways and scoop out the seeds with a teaspoon. Slice the flesh finely and add to the cooled vinegar.

Cook the sushi rice according to packet instructions, then transfer to a bowl, strain the vinegar mixture over it, reserving the cucumber, stir and leave to cool.

Transfer the cooled rice to a large salad bowl and toss gently with the reserved cucumber, salmon, avocado and spring onions. Sprinkle with toasted sesame seeds and serve immediately.

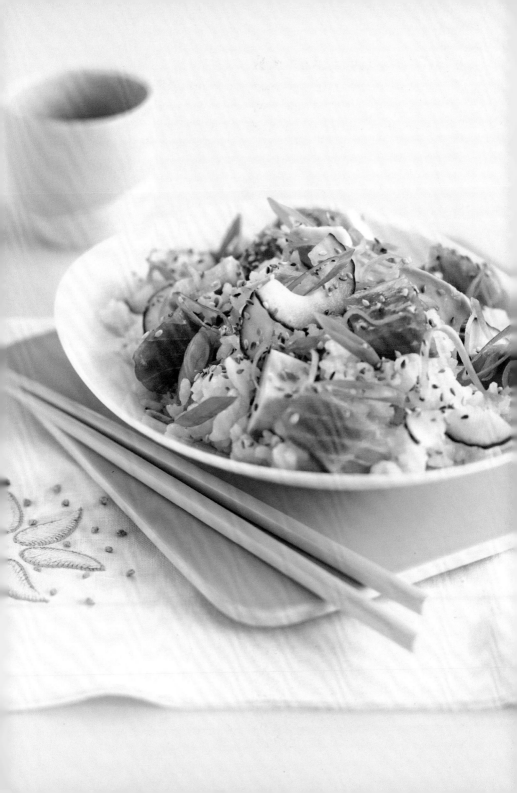

LETTUCE WRAPPERS WITH CRAB

These delicious wrappers are low in saturated fat and calories, but they are guaranteed to lift the mood and assuage hunger.

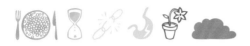

Preparation time: 30 minutes
Serves 4

....

1 cooked **crab**, about 500 g (1 lb)
4 small **Romaine lettuce leaves**,
  hard stalks removed

Cucumber relish
¼ **cucumber**, finely diced
3 **spring onions**, thinly sliced
½ large **red chilli**, deseeded
  and finely chopped
2 tbsps **cider vinegar**
1 tsp **light soy sauce**
1 tsp **caster sugar**
4 tsps finely chopped fresh **coriander**
  or **mint**
sea salt and **black pepper**

To make the relish, mix all the ingredients in a bowl and season to taste.

....

To prepare the crab, twist off the two large claws and the legs. Working on one leg or claw at a time, tap the shell with a rolling pin to break it, then use a small knife or skewer to remove all the white meat inside. Place in a bowl and set aside.

....

Turn the crab body upside-down on a board and press down hard on the undershell until it makes a cracking noise. Use your fingers to separate the top shell from the undershell. Scoop the brown meat from the top shell and place in the bowl with the leg and claw meat.

....

Remove the pointed, spongy lungs from the top of the crab body, then pick all the white meat from the chambers, using a knife or rolling pin to break up the shell as necessary. Place the meat in the bowl and mix the white and brown meat together.

....

When ready to serve, spoon the crab meat on to the lettuce leaves and top with the cucumber relish. Roll up and eat with the fingers.

....

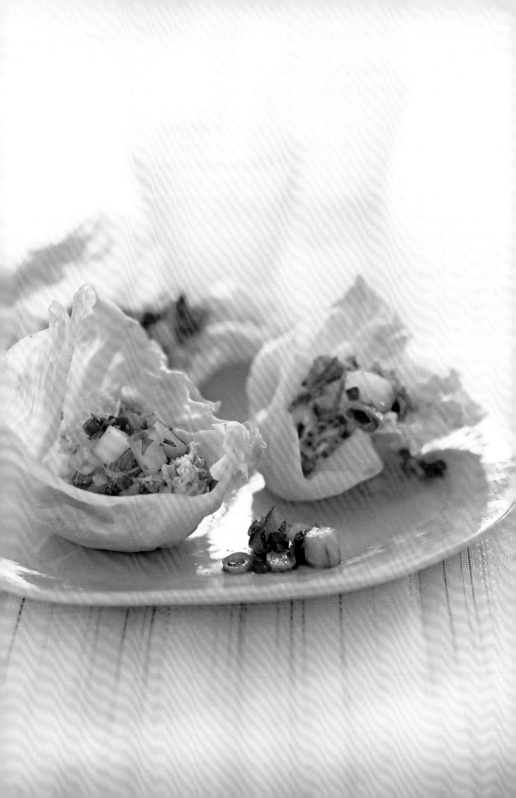

SCALLOP, PARSNIP & CARROT SALAD

This creamy, high fibre salad contains scallops to protect the heart, lower blood pressure, lift mood and satisfy hunger.

Preparation time: 15 minutes
Cooking time: 25 minutes
Serves 4
....

4 unpeeled **carrots**, quartered lengthways
3 unpeeled **parsnips**, quartered lengthways
2 tbsps **olive oil**
1 tbsp **cumin seeds**
12 large **scallops**
2 tbsps **lemon juice**
sea salt and **black pepper**
chopped **parsley**, to garnish

Dressing:
6 tbsps **low-fat live natural yogurt**
2 tbsps **lemon juice**
2 tbsps **olive oil**
1 tsp **ground cumin**

Place the carrots and parsnips on a foil-lined baking sheet, drizzle with half the oil, scatter over the cumin seeds and season to taste. Place in a preheated oven, 180°C (350°F), Gas Mark 4, for 20–25 minutes until tender.

....

Meanwhile, make the dressing. Place all the ingredients in a small bowl, mix well and season to taste.

....

Trim the scallops to remove the tough muscle on the outside of the white fleshy part. Heat the remaining oil in a large frying pan over a high heat and cook the scallops for 2 minutes on each side until just cooked through. Drizzle with the lemon juice and transfer to a large bowl with any cooking juices.

....

Add the carrots and parsnips to the bowl and toss together, then transfer to warmed serving plates. Spoon over the yogurt dressing, garnish with parsley and serve immediately.

....

GREEN BEAN & ASPARAGUS SALAD

This crunchy salad will help to banish tummy fat, control high blood pressure and boost the metabolism.

Preparation time: 10 minutes
Cooking time: 10 minutes
Serves 4
....

200 g (7 oz) fine **green beans**, trimmed
250 g (8 oz) **asparagus**, trimmed
4 **eggs**
5 tbsps **olive oil**
3 tsps **ready-made tapenade**
3 tsps **balsamic vinegar**
100 g (3½ oz) **rocket**
75 g (3 oz) pitted **black olives**
75 g (3 oz) **Parmesan cheese**, shaved
sea salt and **black pepper**

Cook the green beans in a steamer set over a saucepan of gently simmering water for 3 minutes. Add the asparagus and cook for a further 5 minutes until the vegetables are just tender.
....

Meanwhile, place the eggs in a small saucepan, cover with cold water and bring quickly to the boil. Simmer for 2–3 minutes to soft boil, then drain, peel and halve. Mix together the oil, tapenade and vinegar in a small bowl and season to taste.
....

Divide the rocket leaves between 4 serving plates and top with the eggs. Arrange the beans and asparagus around the edge, then drizzle with the dressing. Scatter with the olives and Parmesan shavings and serve immediately.
....

PUMPKIN, FETA & PINE NUT SALAD

Pumpkin is rich in fibre, antioxidants and nutrients to help regulate blood sugar and feta is rich in calcium, to promote relaxation.

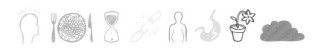

Preparation time: 15 minutes
Cooking time: 25 minutes
Serves 4

500 g (1 lb) **pumpkin**, peeled, deseeded
and cut into 2 cm (¾ inch) cubes
1 tbsp **olive oil**
2 **thyme sprigs**, roughly chopped
200 g (7 oz) **mixed baby salad leaves**
50 g (2 oz) **feta cheese**
sea salt and **black pepper**

Dressing
1 tsp **Dijon mustard**
2 tbsps **balsamic vinegar**
4 tbsps **olive oil**

To serve
2 tbsps **pine nuts**
2 tbsps **pumpkin seeds**

Place the pumpkin in a roasting tin, drizzle with the oil, scatter with the thyme and season to taste. Place in a preheated oven, 190°C (375°F), Gas Mark 5, for 25 minutes or until tender. Allow to cool slightly.

Meanwhile, whisk all the dressing ingredients together and season to taste. Place the pine nuts and pumpkin seeds in a frying pan over a medium heat and dry-fry until lightly toasted.

Place the salad leaves in a large bowl, add the cooked pumpkin and crumble in the feta. Drizzle over the dressing and toss carefully to combine.

Divide the salad between 4 serving plates, sprinkle with the toasted pine nuts and pumpkin seeds and serve immediately.

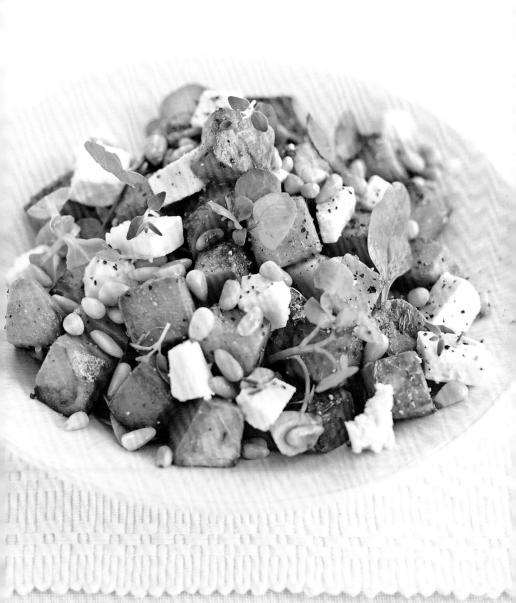

RED PEPPER & FETA ROLLS WITH OLIVES

These tasty, Mediterranean rolls are chock-full of nutrients to support healthy weight loss and leave you looking and feeling great.

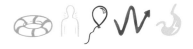

Preparation time: 5 minutes, plus cooling
Cooking time: 10 minutes
Serves 4

2 **red peppers**, cored, deseeded
   and quartered lengthways
100 g (3½ oz) **feta cheese**, crumbled
16 **basil leaves**
16 pitted **black olives**, halved
15 g (½ oz) **pine nuts**, toasted
1 tbsp **ready-made pesto**
1 tbsp **ready-made vinaigrette**

To serve:
100 g (3½ oz) **rocket**
wholemeal crusty bread

Arrange the peppers, skin-side up, on a baking sheet and place under a preheated hot grill for 7–8 minutes until the skins are blackened. Transfer the peppers to a plastic bag, seal the top and leave to cool for 20 minutes, then remove the skins.

Lay the skinned pepper quarters on a board and top with the feta, basil leaves, olives and pine nuts. Carefully roll up the peppers, secure with cocktail sticks and divide between 4 serving plates.

Whisk the pesto with the vinaigrette and drizzle over the pepper rolls. Serve with the rocket and wholemeal crusty bread.

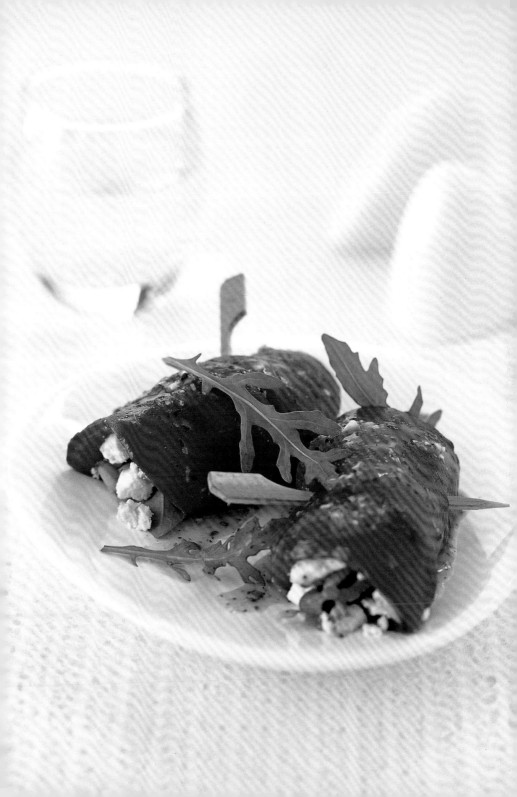

TUNA SKEWERS WITH COCONUT & MANGO SALAD

The fragrance and flavour of these zesty skewers alongside the fresh, antioxidant-rich salad are sublime.

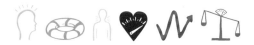

Preparation time: 20 minutes, plus marinating
Cooking time: 5–10 minutes
Serves 4

....

2.5 cm (1 inch) piece of **fresh root ginger**, peeled and finely grated
4 **garlic cloves**, crushed
1 tsp **cayenne pepper**
1 tsp **ground coriander**
1 tsp **ground turmeric**
½ tsp **ground cinnamon**
finely grated rind of 1 **lime**
3 tbsps **olive oil**
625 g (1¼ lb) **tuna steaks**, cubed
sea salt and **black pepper**
chopped fresh **coriander**, to serve

Coconut & mango salad
100 g (3½ oz) **dried coconut flakes**
1 tbsp **olive oil**
2 tsps **honey**
finely grated rind and juice of 1 **lime**
200 g (7 oz) **mixed salad leaves**
2 ripe **mangoes**, peeled, stoned and cubed
1 **avocado**, peeled, stoned and cubed

Place 8 wooden skewers in a bowl of water and leave to soak. Meanwhile, place the ginger in a bowl with the garlic, cayenne pepper, ground coriander, turmeric, cinnamon, lime rind, oil and ½ tsp of salt. Mix well, add the tuna and toss to coat. Cover and marinate in the refrigerator for about an hour.

To make the salad, place the coconut flakes in a dry frying pan over a medium heat and toast for about 4 minutes until just beginning to brown. Allow to cool.

To make the salad dressing, place the olive oil, honey, lime rind and juice in a small bowl, season to taste and mix well.

Thread the tuna on the soaked skewers and place on a foil-lined baking sheet. Brush with the remaining marinade and place under a preheated hot grill for 1–2 minutes on each side, until a little charred on the outside but still pink in the middle.

Place the salad leaves in a large bowl and add the mango, coconut and avocado. Drizzle with the dressing and toss well. Arrange the tuna skewers on serving plates, sprinkle with fresh coriander and serve with the salad.

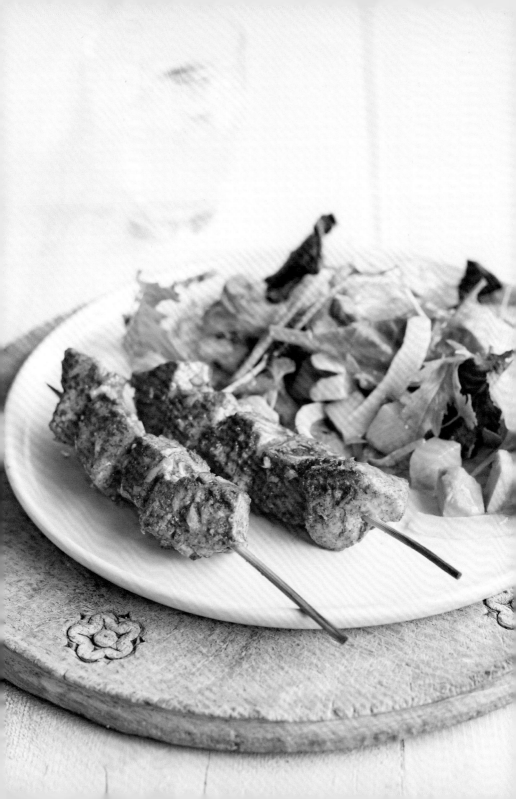

SMOKED HADDOCK WITH POACHED EGGS

Rich in protein to ease hunger and encourage healthy weight loss, this dish is quick to prepare and ideal for busy weeknights.

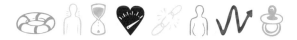

Preparation time: 10 minutes
Cooking time: about 20 minutes
Serves 4
....

750 g (1½ lb) **new potatoes**
4 **spring onions**, sliced
2 tbsps **low-fat crème fraîche**
75 g (3 oz) **watercress**
4 **smoked haddock fillets**,
    about 150 g (5 oz) each
150 ml (¼ pint) **skimmed milk**
1 **bay leaf**
4 **eggs**
sea salt and **black pepper**

Cook the potatoes in a saucepan of lightly salted boiling water for 12–15 minutes until tender. Drain, lightly crush with a fork, then stir in the spring onions, crème fraîche and watercress and season to taste. Keep warm.

Meanwhile, place the fish and milk in a large frying pan with the bay leaf. Bring to the boil over a medium heat, then cover and simmer for 5–6 minutes until the fish is cooked through.

Bring a large saucepan of water to a gentle simmer. Carefully break 2 eggs into the water and cook for 3 minutes until the whites are just set. Remove with a slotted spoon and keep warm while cooking the remaining eggs.

Divide the potatoes between 4 serving plates and arrange the haddock on top. Top with the poached eggs and a sprinkling of black pepper and serve immediately.

BAKED FISH WITH LEMON GRASS & GREEN PAPAYA SALAD

This Thai-inspired dish is low in calories and high in slimming power, with heart-supporting omega-3 oils.

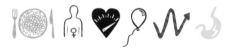

Preparation time: 25 minutes
Cooking time: 20–25 minutes
Serves 4
················

4 whole **fish**, about 250 g (8 oz each),
     such as sea bream, red snapper or
     mackerel, gutted and scaled
4 **lemon grass stalks**,
     cut into 2.5 cm (1 inch) lengths
2 unpeeled **carrots**, cut into matchsticks
1½ tbsps **light soy sauce**, plus extra to serve
2 tbsps **lime juice**

To serve
small handful of chopped fresh **coriander**
1 **red chilli**, deseeded and sliced
lemon wedges

Green papaya salad
2 **garlic cloves**, peeled
100 g (3½ oz) **roasted peanuts**
400 g (13 oz) **green papaya**,
     peeled and finely shredded
100 g (3½ oz) **green beans**,
     cut into 2.5 cm (1 inch) lengths
2 tsps **dried shrimp paste**
2 small **bird's eye chillies**, finely chopped
2 tbsps clear **honey**
1 tbsp **Thai fish sauce**
finely grated rind and juice of 1 **lime**
8 **cherry tomatoes**

Place the fish in an ovenproof dish and use a sharp knife to score each side 3 or 4 times. Sprinkle with the lemon grass, carrots, soy sauce and lime juice. Cover with foil and place in a preheated oven, 180°C (350°F), Gas Mark 4, for 20–25 minutes or until a skewer can be inserted into the flesh without resistance.

·······································

Meanwhile, make the salad with a large pestle and mortar. Place the garlic in the mortar and pound to break it up. Add the peanuts and pound roughly. Add the papaya and pound softly, using a spoon to scrape down the sides, turning and mixing well.

·······································

Add the green beans and shrimp paste and keep pounding and turning to soften the beans. Add the chilli, honey, fish sauce, lime juice and rind and lightly pound together for another minute. Add the tomatoes and lightly pound for another minute. Taste and add more honey, fish sauce, lime juice or chilli if necessary – it should be a balance of sweet, sour, salty and hot.

·······································

Place the fish on warmed serving plates and spoon over the cooking juices. Sprinkle with chopped coriander and sliced chilli and serve with the green papaya salad, lemon wedges and a small bowl of soy sauce.

·······································

CHICKEN BROCHETTES WITH CUCUMBER & KELP SALAD

A delicious combination of thyroid- and metabolism-boosting kelp with marinated, grilled chicken.

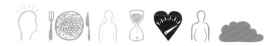

Preparation time: 20 minutes, plus soaking and marinating
Cooking time: 10 minutes
Serves 4
....

1 tbsp **olive oil**, plus extra for brushing
finely grated rind and juice of 1 **lime**
2 tsps **dried oregano**
1 tsp **paprika**
4 boneless, skinless **chicken breasts**
sea salt and **black pepper**
wholemeal pitta breads, to serve

Cucumber & kelp salad
50 g (2 oz) **dried kelp**, cut into strips
juice of 1 **lime**
1 large **cucumber**, thinly sliced
1 tbsp **rice vinegar**
½ tsp **cider vinegar**
1 tbsp **sesame oil**
2 tsps **coconut palm sugar**
2 tbsps **toasted sesame seeds**
2 **spring onions**, thinly sliced

At least 10 hours before you wish to serve this dish, place the kelp in a large bowl with the lime juice and enough water to cover and set aside to soak. If the water has been fully absorbed after 3–4 hours, add more to cover again. The kelp will expand to about 5 times its original size.

Meanwhile, place the olive oil, lime rind and juice, oregano and paprika in a bowl, season to taste and stir well. Add the chicken and stir to coat, cover and refrigerate for at least 2 hours, stirring again from time to time. Place 4 wooden skewers in a bowl of water and leave to soak.

Rinse and drain the kelp and place in a large bowl with the cucumber, vinegars, oil and sugar, mix well and set aside.

Cut the chicken into bite-size pieces and thread on the skewers. Place the skewers on a foil-lined baking sheet and brush with the remaining marinade. Place under a preheated hot grill for about 5 minutes on each side, brushing with a little olive oil if required, until golden and cooked through.

Stir the sesame seeds and onions into the salad and serve with the chicken brochettes and some wholemeal pitta breads.

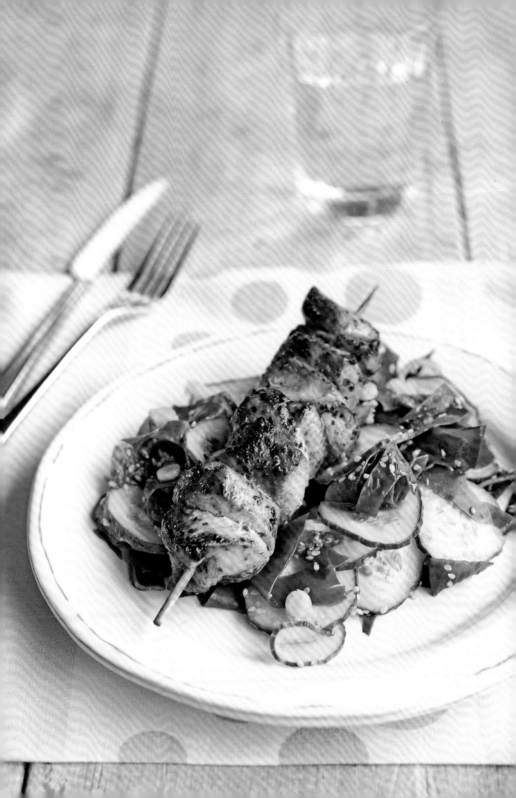

CHICKEN & BLUEBERRY PASTA SALAD

This filling salad will not only keep you going through the evening, but will encourage restful sleep as well.

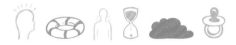

Preparation time: 10 minutes
Cooking time: 20 minutes
Serves 4
....

4 boneless, skinless **chicken breasts**
finely grated rind and juice of 2 **limes**
2 tbsps chopped **thyme**
200 g (7 oz) **wholemeal** or **spelt penne**
3 tbsps **olive oil**
3 **shallots**, peeled and diced
100 ml (3½ fl oz) **chicken stock**
100 g (3½ oz) **feta cheese**, crumbled
100 g (3½oz) **blueberries**
2 **celery sticks**, finely chopped
100 g (3½ oz) **rocket**
sea salt and **black pepper**

Place the chicken breasts in a large saucepan and cover with water. Add half the lime rind and half the thyme and bring to the boil over a medium heat. Reduce the heat and simmer gently for about 10 minutes, or until just cooked through. Drain and allow to cool a little.

Meanwhile, cook the pasta in a saucepan of lightly salted boiling water according to packet instructions until tender but still with a little bite. Drain and place in a large bowl.

Heat the oil in a saucepan over a medium heat, add the shallots and cook for 2–3 minutes, or until softened. Stir in the stock, half the feta and the lime juice, and cook until the feta melts into the stock.

Pour the sauce over the pasta in the bowl, then add the blueberries, celery and the remaining lime rind and thyme. Season to taste, crumble in the remaining feta and toss together to combine.

Arrange the rocket on a large platter and top with the pasta. Serve warm or cold.

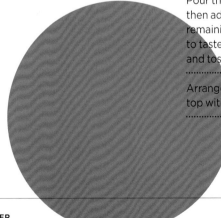

CHICKEN & APPLE STEW

This winning combination of nutty buckwheat, warming spices and fresh apples balances blood sugar and encourages a good night's sleep.

Preparation time: 20 minutes
Cooking time: 50 minutes
Serves 4

125 g (4 oz) **buckwheat**
2 tbsps **olive oil**
75 g (3 oz) **almonds**, chopped
1 tsp **cinnamon**
1 tsp **allspice**
1 tsp **ground cumin**
1 tsp **ground cardamom**
2 large **onions**, thinly sliced
4 large boneless, skinless **chicken thighs**
3 **cooking apples**, cored and
　cut into chunks
2 tsps chopped **thyme**
2 tbsps **cider vinegar**
3 tbsps **cider**
300 ml (½ pint) **chicken stock**
sea salt and **black pepper**
green salad, to serve

Cook the buckwheat in a saucepan of lightly salted boiling water according to packet instructions until tender. Drain and set aside.

Meanwhile, heat half the oil in a large frying pan or wok over a medium heat. Add the almonds and spices, season to taste and cook until the almonds are well coated and beginning to caramelize. Tip into a bowl and set aside.

Heat the remaining oil in the frying pan over a low heat and add the onions. Cook for about 15 minutes until very soft and beginning to colour. Add the chicken and cook for 5 minutes, until lightly browned all over. Add the apples and cook for a further 5 minutes, then stir in the thyme.

Add the cider vinegar, cider and stock, increase the heat and bring to the boil. Reduce the heat and simmer for about 20 minutes until the chicken is cooked through and the apples are beginning to break up.

Stir in the buckwheat and almonds, season to taste and warm through. Serve in warmed bowls with a green salad.

ROMAN CHICKEN WITH PEPPERS

Bursting with Mediterranean flavours and packed with fibre and chromium, this tasty chicken dish will leave you feeling satisfied.

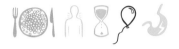

Preparation time: 15 minutes
Cooking time: 30 minutes
Serves 4
....

3 tbsps **olive oil**
4 boneless, skinless **chicken breasts**
1 **red onion**, sliced
3 **garlic cloves**, finely chopped
2 **red peppers**, cored, deseeded and sliced
1 **yellow pepper**, cored, deseeded and sliced
1 **green pepper**, cored, deseeded and sliced
100 g (3½ oz) **button mushrooms**
125 g (4 oz) **pitted green olives**
400 g (13 oz) can **cherry tomatoes**
300 ml (½ pint) **chicken stock**
2 **oregano sprigs**
2 tbsps chopped **parsley**
sea salt and **black pepper**
brown rice, to serve

Heat the oil in large, heavy-based saucepan over a high heat, add the chicken and brown all over. Remove from the pan and set aside.
....

Add the onion and garlic to the pan and cook for 1–2 minutes. Add the peppers and mushrooms and cook for a further 2–3 minutes, then add the olives, cherry tomatoes, stock and oregano.
....

Return the chicken to the pan, cover and bring to the boil. Reduce the heat and simmer for about 20 minutes until the chicken is cooked through. Stir in the parsley, season to taste and serve with a little brown rice.
....

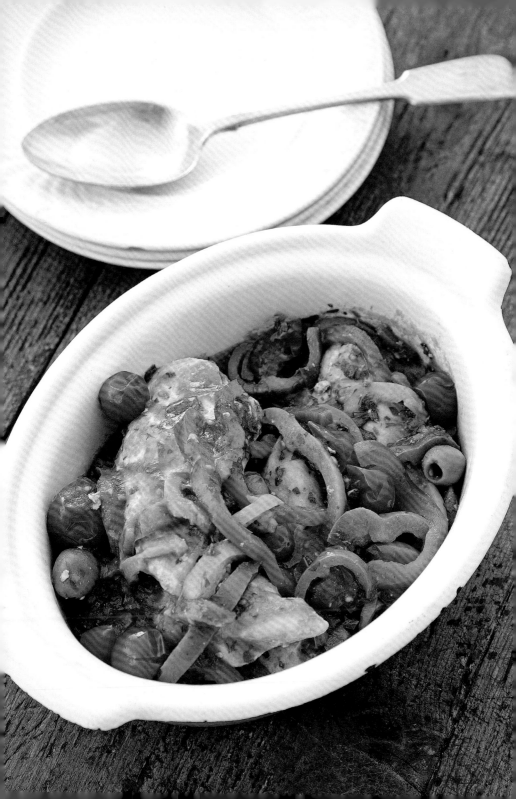

LAMB & APRICOT TAGINE WITH PEARL BARLEY

Fragrant and tasty, this tagine contains a host of nutrients to balance hormones, boost mood and kick-start the metabolism.

Preparation time: 15 minutes
Cooking time: 1¼ hours
Serves 4

olive oil spray
625 g (1¼ lb) lean diced **lamb**
1 **red onion**, chopped
1 unpeeled **carrot**, chopped
1 tsp **paprika**
1 tsp **ground coriander**
1 tsp **fennel seeds**
3 cm (1¼ inch) **cinnamon stick**
2 **garlic cloves**, crushed
2 **bay leaves**
3 tbsps **lime juice**
750 ml (1¼ pints) **chicken stock**
75 g (3 oz) soft **dried apricots**
400 g (13 oz) can **chopped tomatoes**
65 g (2½ oz) **pearl barley**
15 g (½ oz) chopped fresh **coriander**,
    plus extra to garnish
200 g (7 oz) **couscous**
sea salt and **black pepper**

Heat a large heavy-based saucepan over a high heat, spray lightly with oil and cook the lamb briefly, in batches if necessary, until browned all over. Remove from the pan with a slotted spoon and set aside.

Add the onion and carrot to the pan and cook briefly until golden. Return the lamb to the pan, stir in the spices, garlic, bay leaves, two-thirds of the lime juice, the stock, apricots, tomatoes and barley.

Season to taste, cover and bring to the boil. Reduce the heat and simmer for 1 hour or until the lamb is tender. Stir in the coriander and remaining lime juice.

Meanwhile, prepare the couscous according to packet instructions. Serve the hot tagine with the couscous, garnished with fresh coriander.

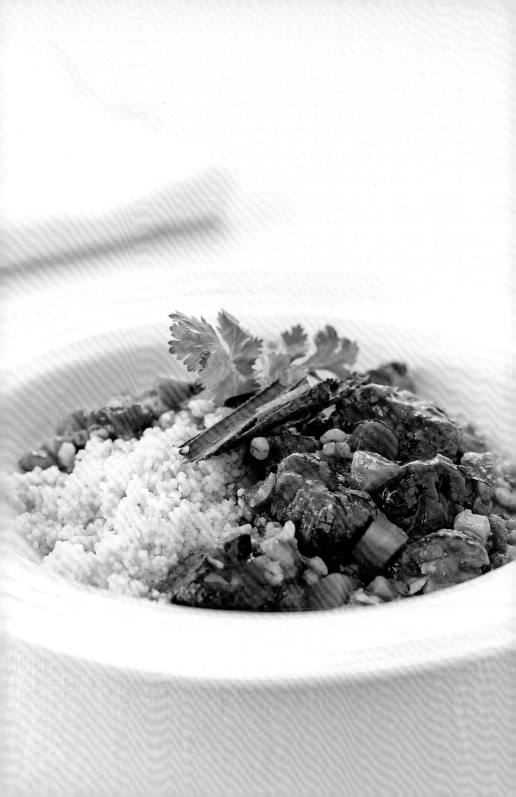

CHEESY PORK WITH PARSNIP PURÉE

Bound to satisfy even the heartiest appetite, these lean, cheesy pork steaks are deliciously creamy and moreish.

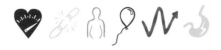

Preparation time: 15 minutes
Cooking time: 20 minutes
Serves 4

....

4 **lean pork loin steaks**,
   about 125 g (4 oz) each
1 tsp **olive oil**
50 g (2 oz) **Wensleydale**
   or **Cheshire cheese**, crumbled
½ tbsp chopped **sage**
75 g (3 oz) **wholemeal breadcrumbs**
1 **egg yolk**, beaten
625 g (1¼ lb) unpeeled **parsnips**, chopped
2 **garlic cloves**, peeled
3 tbsps **low-fat crème fraîche**
sea salt and **black pepper**
steamed **green beans**, to serve

Season the pork steaks with a little salt and plenty of pepper. Heat the oil in a nonstick frying pan over a high heat, add the pork steaks and fry for 2 minutes on each side until browned, then transfer to an ovenproof dish.

....

Place the cheese in a bowl with the sage, breadcrumbs and egg yolk. Mix well and divide the mixture into 4 portions. Use to top the pork steaks, pressing down gently. Place in a preheated oven, 200°C (400°F), Gas Mark 6, for 12–15 minutes until the topping is golden and the pork is cooked through.

....

Meanwhile, cook the parsnips and garlic in a saucepan of lightly salted boiling water for 10–12 minutes until tender. Drain and mash with the crème fraîche and plenty of pepper. Serve with the pork steaks and some steamed green beans.

....

SLOW-COOKED SPICY BEEF

Meltingly tender beef with warming, digestion-boosting, fat-burning spices – this is a hearty meal in a bowl.

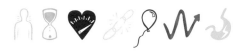

Preparation time: 20 minutes
Cooking time: 2¼ hours
Serves 4–6
....

1 tbsp **groundnut oil**
1 large **onion**, chopped
750 g (1½ lb) **stewing steak**, cubed
2 tbsps **tomato purée**
3 **tomatoes**, chopped
250 ml (8 fl oz) **water**
3 tbsps **low-fat live natural yogurt**,
  plus extra to serve
1 tsp **nigella seeds**
sea salt and **black pepper**
wholemeal naan bread, to serve

Spice paste
2 tsps **cumin seeds**
1 tsp **coriander seeds**
½ tsp **fennel seeds**
1 tsp **ground cinnamon**
2 **garlic cloves**, chopped
1 tbsp grated **fresh root ginger**
1–2 small **green chillies**
1 tsp **paprika**
1 tsp **ground turmeric**
2 tbsps **tomato purée**
2 tbsps **groundnut oil**
25 g (1 oz) **coriander** leaves,
  plus extra to garnish

To make the spice paste, dry-fry the cumin, coriander and fennel in a small frying pan over a medium heat for 2–3 minutes until fragrant. Tip the contents of the pan into a mini blender and blend to a fine powder. Add the remaining spice paste ingredients and blend until smooth.

....

Heat the oil in a large saucepan over a medium heat, add the onion and cook for 5–6 minutes or until beginning to colour, stirring occasionally. Add 3 tbsps of the spice paste and stir-fry for 1–2 minutes.

....

Stir in the meat and cook for 4–5 minutes or until the meat is browned and well coated. Stir in the tomato purée, tomatoes, measurement water and yogurt, and bring to the boil. Reduce the heat, cover and simmer for 2 hours or until tender, adding more liquid if necessary.

....

Season to taste and ladle into warmed bowls. Sprinkle with the nigella seeds and garnish with coriander leaves. Serve hot with naan bread and yogurt.

....

MOROCCAN CHICKPEAS WITH CARROTS & DATES

This meal is bursting with nutrients that support weight loss and, most importantly, it's delicious and satisfying.

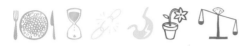

Preparation time: 10 minutes
Cooking time: 30 minutes
Serves 4
....

1 tbsp **olive oil**
2 large **onions**, sliced
2 **garlic cloves**, sliced
2 large unpeeled **carrots**, sliced
1 large unpeeled **parsnip**, sliced
4 tsps **ground cumin**
2 tsps **ground turmeric**
1 tsp **ground cinnamon**, plus extra to serve
2.5 cm (1 inch) piece of **fresh root ginger**,
      peeled and finely grated
250 ml (8 fl oz) **vegetable stock**
2 x 400 g (13 oz) cans **chopped tomatoes**
2 x 400 g (13 oz) cans **chickpeas**,
      rinsed and drained
100 g (3½ oz) **dried dates**,
      pitted and coarsely chopped
1 tbsp **honey**
finely grated rind and juice of ½ **lemon**
sea salt and **black pepper**

To serve
50 g (2 oz) **flaked almonds**, lightly toasted
25 g (1 oz) fresh **coriander**, chopped

Heat the oil in a large, heavy-based saucepan over a medium heat and add the onions. Cook for 5–10 minutes until soft and starting to colour. Add the garlic and cook for 1 minute more, then stir n the carrots and parsnip.

....

Add the cumin, turmeric, cinnamon and ginger and mix well to coat the vegetables. Pour in the stock and tomatoes and bring to the boil.
....

Add the chickpeas and dates, reduce the heat and simmer, uncovered, for about 15 minutes until the vegetables are tender.
....

Add the honey, lemon rind and juice and season to taste. Serve in warmed bowls, sprinkled with the almonds, fresh coriander and a little extra cinnamon.
....

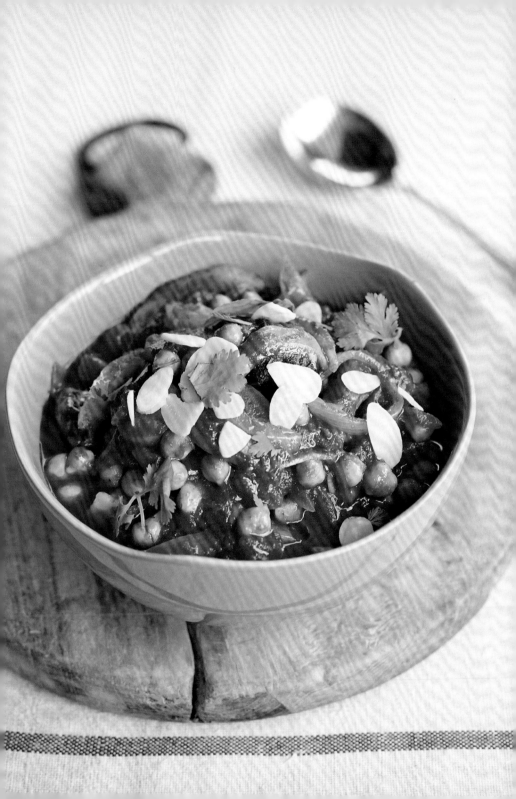

VEGETABLE & TOFU STIR-FRY

The tofu in this quick and easy supper dish is rich in phytoestrogens to help balance hormones.

     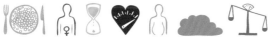

Preparation time: 15 minutes
Cooking time: 10 minutes
Serves 4
....

3 tbsps **sunflower oil**
300 g (10 oz) **firm tofu**, cubed
1 **onion**, sliced
2 unpeeled **carrots**, sliced
150 g (5 oz) **broccoli**, cut into small florets
1 **red pepper**, cored, deseeded and sliced
1 large **courgette**, sliced
150 g (5 oz) **sugar snap peas**
2 tbsps **dark soy sauce**
2 tbsps **sweet chilli sauce**
125 ml (4 fl oz) **water**

To garnish
chopped **red chillies**
Thai basil leaves

Heat 1 tbsp of the oil in a wok or large frying pan until starting to smoke, add the tofu and stir-fry over a high heat for 2 minutes or until golden all over. Remove with a slotted spoon and keep warm.

Heat the remaining oil in the pan, add the onion and carrots and stir-fry for 1½ minutes. Add the broccoli and red pepper and stir-fry for 1 minute, then add the courgette and sugar snap peas and stir-fry for 1 minute.

Mix together the soy and chilli sauces and measurement water and add to the pan with the tofu. Cook for 1 minute more. Serve in warmed bowls, garnished with chopped red chillies and Thai basil leaves.

PUMPKIN CURRY WITH PINK GRAPEFRUIT SALAD

This tasty curry is rich in antioxidants to support general health and helps combat the symptoms of stress, including low energy.

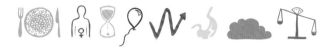

Preparation time: 20 minutes
Cooking time: 25 minutes
Serves 4

1 tbsp **olive oil**
1 large **onion**, finely chopped
2 **garlic cloves**, finely chopped
1 tsp **ground coriander**
1 tsp **ground cumin**
2 tsps **ground turmeric**
1 tsp **curry powder**
1 cm (½ inch) piece of **fresh root ginger**, peeled and finely grated
1 tsp **black mustard seeds**
750 ml (1¼ pints) **vegetable stock**
200 ml (7 fl oz) can **low-fat coconut milk**
750 g (1½ lb) **pumpkin**, peeled, deseeded and cut into chunks
sea salt and **black pepper**
25 g (1 oz) fresh **coriander**, chopped, to serve

Pink grapefruit salad
4 **pink grapefruit**
1 tbsp **olive oil**
2 **spring onions**, finely chopped
1 tbsp **honey**
finely grated rind and juice of ½ **lime**
50 g (2 oz) **mint** leaves
50 g (2 oz) **almonds**, lightly toasted and chopped
50 g (2 oz) fresh **coriander**, chopped

Heat the olive oil in a large saucepan over a medium heat and add the onion. Cook for about 5 minutes until softened, then add the garlic and cook for a further 2 minutes.

Add the ground coriander, cumin, turmeric, curry powder, ginger and mustard seeds, stir well to combine, then pour in the stock and coconut milk. Bring to the boil and add the pumpkin. Reduce the heat and simmer, covered, for 10 minutes until the pumpkin is tender.

Meanwhile, prepare the salad by peeling the grapefruit with a sharp knife. Holding the grapefruit over a bowl to catch the juices, remove the segments by cutting between the membranes with the knife. Arrange the segments on a serving plate and set aside.

Place the oil, spring onions, honey and lime rind and juice in the bowl with the grapefruit juice, season to taste and mix well. Drizzle over the grapefruit segments and sprinkle with the mint, almonds and coriander.

Uncover the curry and cook for a further 4–5 minutes to thicken the sauce. Sprinkle with the coriander and serve with the pink grapefruit salad.

THAI RED VEGETABLE CURRY

A spicy, creamy curry to lift mood, boost energy, balance blood sugar, aid digestion and enhance the metabolism. For an extra boost, serve this curry with coconut rice.

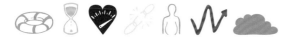

Preparation time: 20 minutes, plus standing
Cooking time: 1 hour
Serves 4
....

1 tbsp **groundnut oil**, plus extra for greasing
1 large **onion**, chopped
100 g (3½ oz) **sweet potato**, peeled and cut into chunks
100 g (3½ oz) **butternut squash**, peeled, deseeded and cut into chunks
400 ml (14 fl oz) can **low-fat coconut milk**
200 ml (7 fl oz) **vegetable stock**
2 large **courgettes**, cut into chunks
100 g (3½ oz) **green beans**, trimmed
400 g (13 oz) can **chickpeas**
200 g (7 oz) can **green lentils**
handful of fresh **coriander**, to serve
plain or **coconut rice**, to serve

Curry paste
2 tsps **cumin seeds**
2 tsps **coriander seeds**
1 tsp **ground turmeric**
3 **red chillies**, deseeded
5 **spring onions**, chopped
2 **garlic cloves**, chopped
2.5 cm (1 inch) piece of **fresh root ginger**, peeled and chopped
4 **lemon grass stalks**, outer leaves discarded, cores chopped
finely grated rind and juice of 1 **lime**
1 tbsp **honey**

To make the spice paste, dry-fry the cumin and coriander seeds in a small frying pan over a medium heat for 2–3 minutes until fragrant. Tip the contents of the pan into a mini blender and blend to a fine powder. Add the remaining curry paste ingredients and blend until smooth, adding a little water if necessary. Season with salt and pepper.
....

Heat the groundnut oil in a large saucepan over a medium heat, add the onion and cook for about 5 minutes until just beginning to soften. Add 3–4 heaped tbsps of the curry paste and cook for about 5 minutes more, until fragrant.
....

Add the sweet potato and squash and stir to coat, then pour in the coconut milk and stock. Bring to the boil, reduce the heat and simmer for about 10 minutes until the vegetables are almost tender.
....

Add the courgettes, green beans and the rinsed and drained chickpeas and lentils and cook for a further 10 minutes until the courgettes are just cooked.
....

Sprinkle with chopped fresh coriander and serve with rice. To make coconut rice, substitute a can of low-fat coconut milk for some of the cooking water.
....

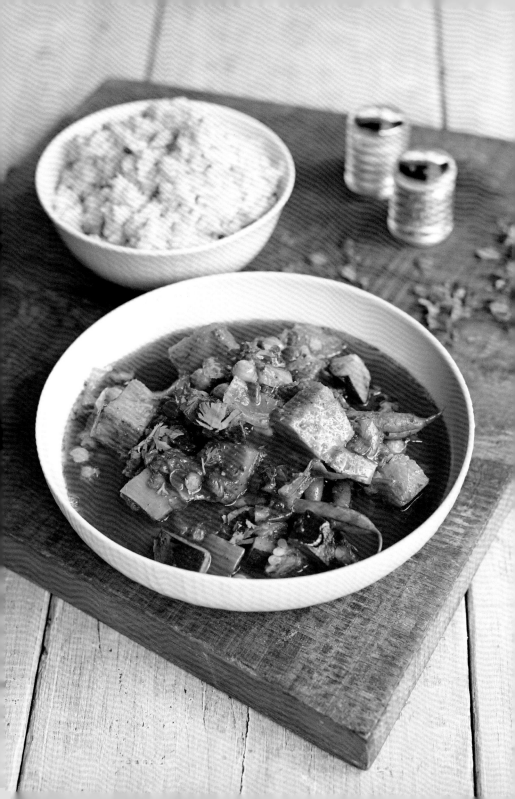

CHOCOLATE ESPRESSO POTS

Dark chocolate boosts energy, balances mood and reduces cravings. These pots do contain saturated fat, though, so save them for a treat.

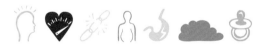

Preparation time: 5 minutes, plus chilling
Cooking time: 5 minutes
Serves 4

....

125 g (4 oz) **plain dark chocolate**, broken into small pieces
2 tsps **instant espresso powder**
150 ml (¼ pint) **double cream**
175 ml (6 fl oz) **low-fat live Greek yogurt**
4 **dark chocolate-coated coffee beans**, to decorate

Place 4 espresso cups or ramekins in the refrigerator to chill. Meanwhile, place the chocolate, espresso powder and 3 tbsps of the cream in a heatproof bowl set over a saucepan of gently simmering water, making sure the water does not touch the bottom of the bowl.

....

Heat, stirring from time to time, until the chocolate has melted. Remove from the heat, stir in the remaining cream and half the yogurt and pour into the chilled cups or ramekins.

....

Spoon the remaining yogurt on top and decorate each portion with a coffee bean. Chill in the refrigerator for at least 10 minutes before serving.

....

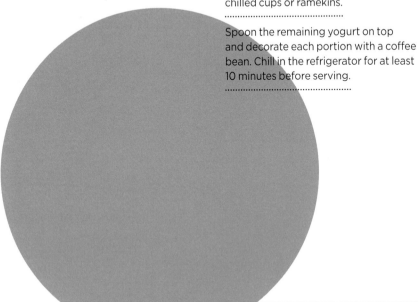

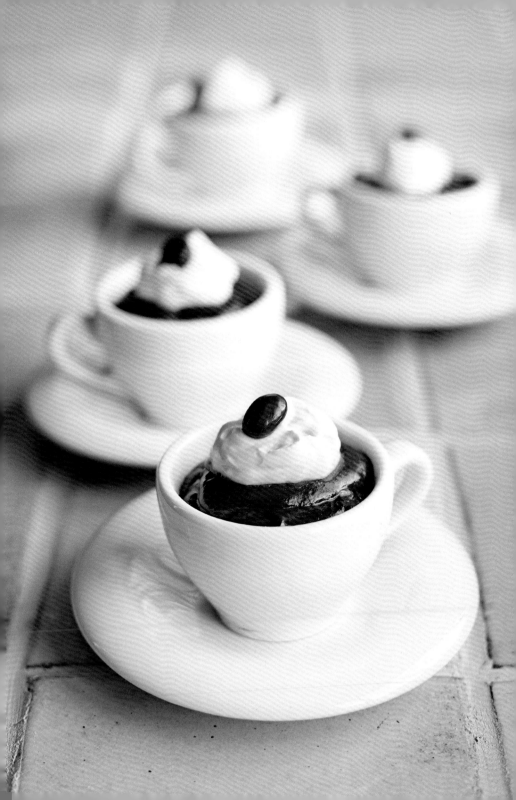

CHOCOLATE-DIPPED CHERRIES

Cherries are wonderful for boosting metabolism and lifting mood; they are particularly delicious with dark chocolate.

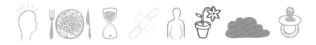

Preparation time: 10 minutes, plus setting
Cooking time: 5 minutes
Serves 4-6
·················

100 g (3½ oz) **plain dark chocolate**, broken into small pieces
200 g (7 oz) **cherries** with stems, rinsed and dried

Place the chocolate in a heatproof bowl set over a saucepan of gently simmering water, making sure the water does not touch the bottom of the bowl. Heat, stirring from time to time, until the chocolate has melted. Remove the bowl from the heat and allow to cool slightly.
···

Hold the cherries by their stems one by one and dip into the chocolate, swirling them a little to get an even coverage. Transfer to a tray lined with baking paper and leave for 10–20 minutes to set.
···

ALMOND & APPLE CAKE WITH VANILLA YOGURT

This cake is bursting with nutrients that encourage weight loss. A little goes a long way, so serve in small portions.

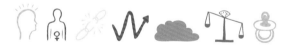

Preparation time: 20 minutes, plus cooling
Cooking time: about 1 hour
Makes 16 slices

200 g (7 oz) **butter**, softened,
    plus extra for greasing
4 **Granny Smith apples**, peeled,
    cored and cut into chunks
200 g (7 oz) **golden caster sugar**
3 large **eggs**, beaten
3–4 tbsps **apple juice**
150 g (5 oz) **self-raising wholemeal flour**
75 g (3 oz) **ground almonds**

To serve
500 g (1 lb) **low-fat live Greek yogurt**
a few drops of **vanilla extract**

Grease a 20 cm (8 inch) round cake tin and line the base with baking paper.

Melt 1 tbsp of the butter in a large saucepan over a medium heat and stir in the apples. Cook for about 5 minutes until softened but still maintaining their shape. Remove from the heat and allow to cool.

Place the remaining butter and the sugar in a large bowl and beat until light and fluffy. Stir in the eggs, one at a time, beating constantly, then add the apple juice.

Sift the flour into the bowl, then add the bran out of the sieve with the ground almonds and half the apples. Fold the ingredients gently to combine.

Smooth the mixture out in the prepared cake tin and top with the remaining apples, pushing them down into the batter so the tops are just showing.

Place in a preheated oven, 180°C (350°F), Gas Mark 4, for 55– 60 minutes until a skewer inserted into the centre of the cake comes out clean. Allow to cool in the tin.

Place the yogurt in a bowl and stir in the vanilla. Serve with the cake.

BLUEBERRY CHEESECAKE POTS

Filled with dairy produce and fat-busting blueberries, these creamy little deconstructed cheesecakes are quick and simple to make.

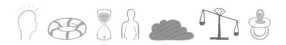

Preparation time: 20 minutes,
    plus cooling and chilling
Cooking time: 5 minutes
Serves 4

200 g (7 oz) **blueberries**
1 tsp **honey**
8 **amaretti biscuits**
25 g (1 oz) **unsalted butter**, melted
150 g (5 oz) **light cream cheese**
150 g (5 oz) **low-fat live Greek yogurt**
4 tbsps **icing sugar**
finely grated rind and juice of 1 **lemon**

Place the blueberries in a small saucepan over a low heat and stir in the honey. Bring to a gentle simmer and cook for about 5 minutes until the blueberries are bursting and their juices running. Remove from the heat and allow to cool.

Place the amaretti biscuits in a food processor and blend to a fine crumb. Add the melted butter and pulse until moist and well combined. Press the mixture into the bottoms of 4 individual serving glasses.

Place the cream cheese, yogurt, icing sugar and lemon rind and juice in a bowl and beat until fluffy and well combined.

Divide the mixture between the 4 glasses, then top with the blueberry mixture. Chill in the refrigerator for 20–30 minutes before serving.

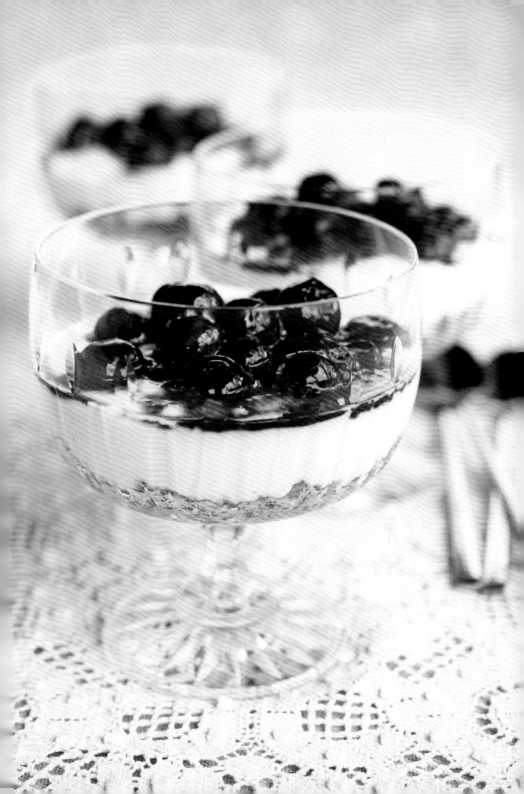

COCONUT MANGO PUDDING

With a host of healthy nutrients, this mango pudding
is utterly delicious, easy to make and surprisingly light.

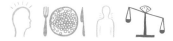

Preparation time: 15 minutes, plus chilling
Cooking time: 2 minutes
Serves 4
....

2 large ripe **mangoes**, peeled,
   stoned and cut into chunks
4 **sheets of gelatine**
125 ml (4 fl oz) hot **water**
6 tbsps **honey**
400 ml (14 fl oz) can **low-fat coconut milk**
mint sprigs, to decorate

Place the mango chunks in a blender
or food processor and blend until
smooth. Place the gelatine sheets
in a small bowl, cover with cold water
and leave to soak for a few minutes.
....

Place the measurement hot water
and honey in a small saucepan over a
medium heat until boiling, then remove
from the heat. Squeeze any excess water
from the gelatine sheets and drop them
into the saucepan, one at a time, stirring
well after each addition to dissolve.
....

Pour the mixture into the blender
or food processor with the mango,
add the coconut milk and blend until
smooth and well combined. Pour into
individual serving glasses and chill in
the refrigerator for about 2 hours until
set. Serve decorated with mint sprigs.
....

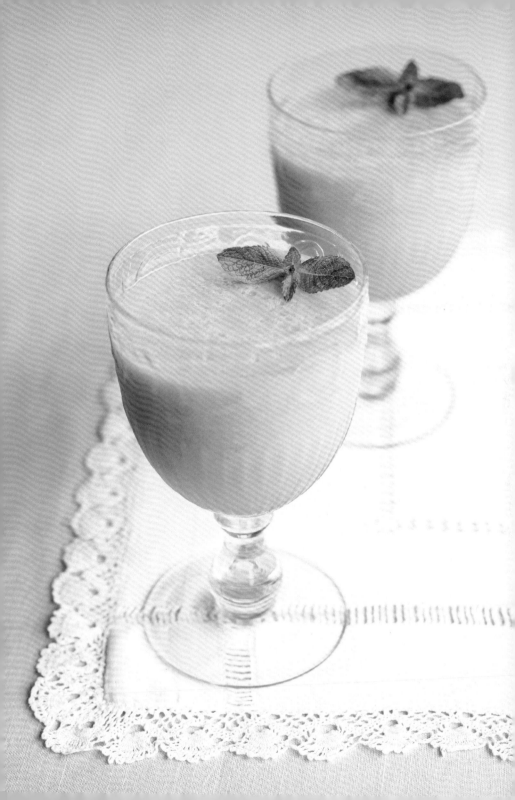

BAKED APPLES

Rich in fibre and packed with crunchy, filling oats and walnuts, this dessert is satisfying and easy to make.

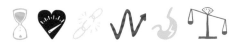

Preparation time: 10 minutes
Cooking time: 25 minutes
Serves 4

....

4 **dessert apples**
5 tbsps **maple syrup**, plus extra for drizzling
75 g (3 oz) **coarse oatmeal** or **steel-cut oats**
50 g (2 oz) **walnuts**, chopped
3 tsps **ground cinnamon**
low-fat live Greek yogurt, to serve

Cut the apples in half lengthways and use a small knife to cut out the cores to leave a cavity in the centre of each apple half. Place the halves, cut-side up, on a baking sheet lined with baking paper.

Place the maple syrup, oatmeal and walnuts in a bowl and stir until well combined. Press the mixture into the cavities in the apples, then sprinkle generously with cinnamon.

Drizzle with a little more maple syrup and place in a preheated oven, 180°C (350°F), Gas Mark 4, for 25 minutes, or until the apples are soft but still holding their shape. Serve warm with Greek yogurt.

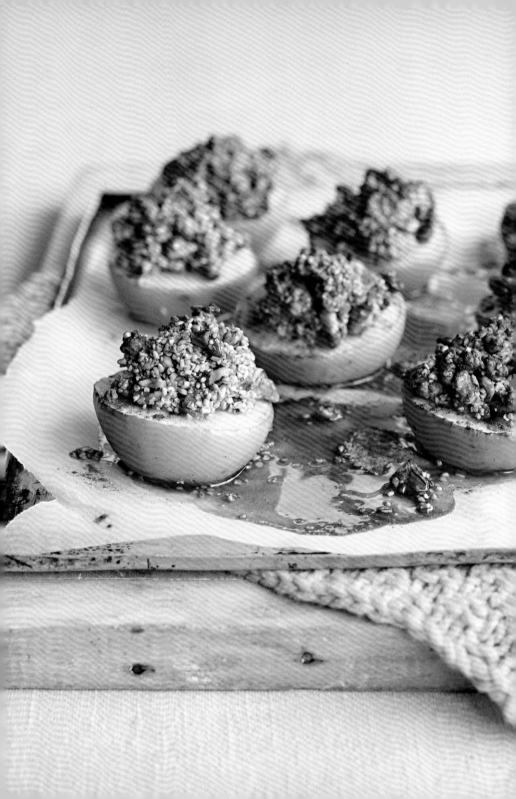

GREEN TEA & GINGER GRANITA

This is a light and refreshing way to end a hearty meal, with warming ginger and antioxidant-rich green tea.

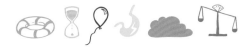

Preparation time: 15 minutes, plus cooling and freezing
Cooking time: 5 minutes
Serves 4

....

750 ml (1¼ pints) **water**
25 g (1 oz) **golden caster sugar**
2 tbsps **honey**
2.5 cm (1 inch) piece of **fresh root ginger**, peeled and finely chopped
5 **green tea bags**
finely grated rind and juice of ½ **orange**

Place the measurement water in a large saucepan over a medium heat, add the sugar, honey, ginger, tea bags and orange rind and stir until the sugar has dissolved. Remove from the heat and allow to cool.

....

Stir in the orange juice, then strain into a shallow tin. Place in the freezer for 30 minutes, then break up the ice crystals with a fork.

....

Freeze for a further 45 minutes and repeat. The granita is ready to serve when it is completely frozen and broken into shards of ice.

....

SLICED ORANGES WITH ALMONDS

This delicious orange salad is high in fibre to balance blood sugar and encourage healthy digestion. Perfect for dessert or breakfast.

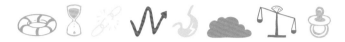

Preparation time: 10 minutes
Serves 4
....

8 **oranges**
1 tbsp **icing sugar**
1 tsp **ground cinnamon**
75 g (3 oz) **almonds**, chopped

Peel 7 of the oranges with a sharp knife, removing most of the white pith with the rind. Slice the oranges into 1 cm (½ inch) thick rounds and arrange on a serving plate.
....

Sprinkle with the icing sugar and drizzle with the rind and juice of the remaining orange Sprinkle with the cinnamon and almonds and serve immediately.
....

GRIDDLED PEACHES & APRICOTS WITH HONEY YOGURT

Rich in antioxidants and fibre, these fragrant fruits are softened and lightly caramelized on a griddle for an unctuous dessert.

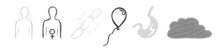

Preparation time: 10 minutes
Cooking time: about 5 minutes
Serves 4

2 tbsps **vanilla sugar**
3 **peaches**, quartered and stoned
4 **apricots**, halved and stoned
200 g (7 oz) **low-fat live Greek yogurt**
2 tbsps clear **honey**

Place the sugar in a large bowl, add the fruit and toss gently to coat.

Preheat a griddle pan until hot, then add the peaches, cut-side down. Cook over a medium heat for 2–3 minutes until caramelized, then add the apricots. Turn over the peaches and cook for a further 2–3 minutes until all the fruit is soft.

Meanwhile, place the yogurt in a bowl and pour over the honey. Stir briefly to create a rippled effect. Serve the warmed griddled fruit with the honey yogurt.

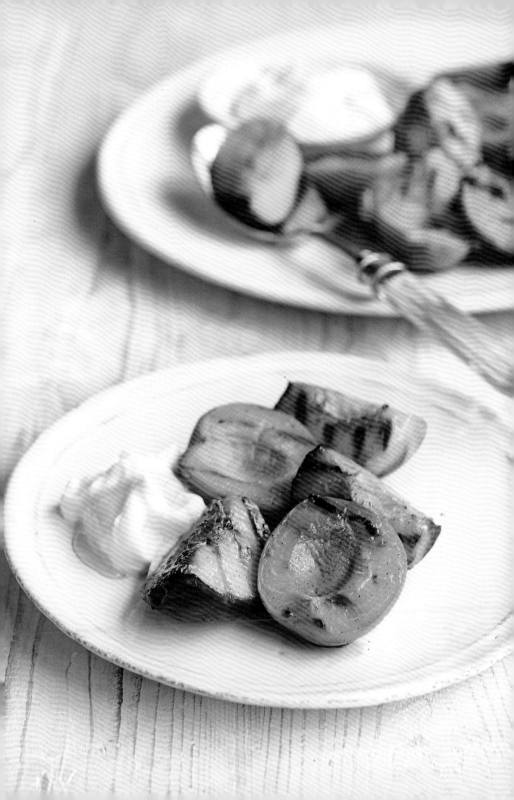

CINNAMON BRIOCHE WITH MIXED BERRIES

These fried slices of eggy brioche are a little sinful, but happily balanced by antioxidant- and fibre-rich berries.

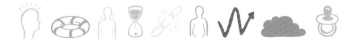

Preparation time: 10 minutes
Cooking time: 10 minutes
Serves 4

1 large **egg**
2 tsps **ground cinnamon**
2 tbsps **golden caster sugar**
125 ml (4 fl oz) **skimmed milk**
1 tbsp **olive oil**
4 slices of **brioche bread**
400 g (13 oz) **mixed berries**, such as strawberries, raspberries, blueberries, redcurrants and blackcurrants
low-fat frozen yogurt, to serve

Place the egg, cinnamon and sugar in a shallow dish, whisk to combine then whisk in the milk.

Heat a large frying pan over a medium heat and add half the olive oil. Dip 2 slices of brioche in the egg mixture, turning to coat evenly, then place in the hot pan. Cook for 2–3 minutes on each side until golden.

Remove the cooked brioche from the pan and keep warm. Repeat with the remaining slices, adding a little more oil if necessary.

Top the brioche with the mixed berries and serve with scoops of frozen yogurt.

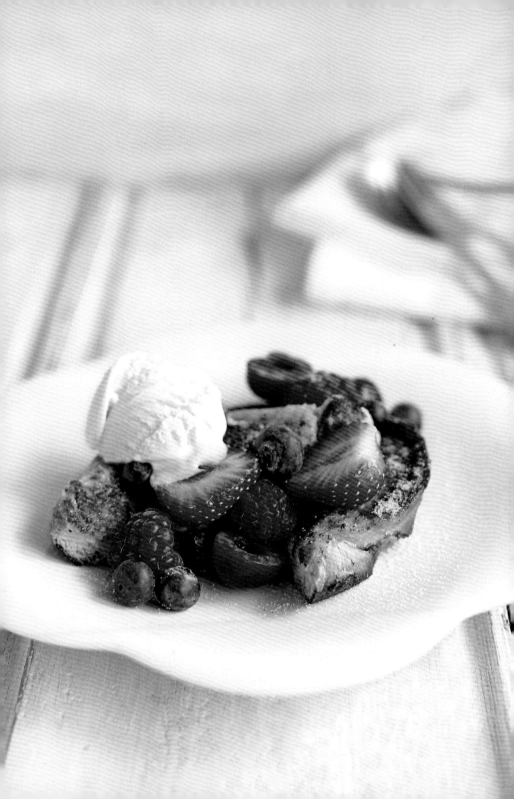

RESOURCES

Action on Addiction
Tel: 0300 330 0659
Email: action@actiononaddiction.org.uk
Website: www.actiononaddiction.org.uk

**British Association for Counselling
and Psychotherapy**
Tel: 0870 443 5252
Website: www.bacp.co.uk

Blood Pressure UK
Tel: 0845 241 0989
Website: www.bloodpressureuk.org

British Heart Foundation
Helpline: 020 7935 0185
Website: www.bhf.org.uk

British Meditation Society
Tel: 01460 62921
Website: www.britishmeditationsociety.org

British Nutrition Foundation
Tel: 020 7557 7930
Email: postbox@nutrition.org.uk
Website: www.nutrition.org.uk

British Thyroid Foundation
Tel: 01423 709707 or 01423 709448
Website: www.btf-thyroid.org

British Wheel of Yoga
Tel: 01529 306 851
Website: www.bwy.org.uk

Core (Fighting Gut and Liver Disease)
Tel: 020 7486 0341
Email: info@corecharity.org.uk
Website: www.corecharity.org.uk

Depression Alliance
Tel: 0845 1232320
Email: information@depressionalliance.org
Website: www.depressionalliance.org

Diabetes UK
Tel: 0845 120 2960
Email: info@diabetes.org.uk
Website: www.diabetes.org.uk

The Menopause Exchange
Tel: 020 8420 7245
Email: info@menopause-exchange.co.uk
Website: www.menopause-exchange.co.uk

NHS Choices Live Well – health and fitness
Website: www.nhs.uk/LiveWell/Fitness/Pages/
Fitnesshome.aspx

The Nutrition Society
Tel: 020 7602 0228
Email: office@nutsoc.org.uk
Website: www.nutsoc.org.uk

Sleep Matters Insomnia Helpline
Tel: 020 8994 9874 (6pm to 8pm)
Email: info@medicaladvisoryservice.org.uk
Website: www.medicaladvisoryservice.org.uk

Weight Concern
Tel: 020 7679 1853
Email: enquiries@weightconcern.org.uk
Website: www.weightconcern.org.uk

Weightwise
British Dietetic Association
Email: info@bda.uk.com
Website: www.bdaweightwise.com

INDEX

Almonds 18
  almond & apple cake
    with vanilla
    yogurt 113
  sliced oranges with
    almonds 121
apples 17
  almond & apple
    cake with vanilla
    yogurt 113
  apple, cinnamon &
    almond muesli 40
  baked apples 118-19
  chicken & apple
    stew 97
  cranberry & apple
    smoothie 64
apricots
  griddled peaches
    & apricots with
    honey yogurt 122
  lamb & apricot
    tagine with pearl
    barley 100
asparagus
  asparagus with
    smoked salmon 53
  green bean &
    asparagus salad 85
aubergine dip with
  toasted torillas 62

Bananas
  banana & almond
    smoothie 46
  date & banana
    pancakes 42
beans
  black bean
    hummus 60
  black bean soup 70
  black beans 21
  green bean &
    asparagus salad 85
  roasted edamame
    beans 56
beef
  peppered beef with
    salad leaves 78

slow cooked spicy
  beef 103
beer belly 26
berries
  cinnamon brioche
    with mixed
    berries 124
  fruity summer
    milkshake 47
  summer berry
    granola 38
bloating 28
blood sugar
  fluctuations 27
blueberries 12
  blueberry cheesecake
    pots 114
  chicken & blueberry
    pasta salad 96
  green tea porridge
    with blueberries 36
broccoli, scallop &,
  broth 68
butternut squash,
  rosemary and
  lentil soup 77

Carrots 16
  Moroccan chickpeas
    with carrots &
    dates 104
  scallop, parsnip
    & carrot salad 84
  spicy carrot & lemon
    soup 76
cheese 25
  cheesy pork with
    parsnip puree 102
  pumpkin, feta & pine
    nut salad 86
  red pepper & feta rolls
    with olives 88
cherries
  chocolate dipped
    cherries 112
chicken 23
  chicken & apple
    stew 97
  chicken & blueberry
    pasta salad 96

chicken brochettes
  with cucumber &
  kelp salad 94
  Roman chicken
    with peppers 98
chickpeas
  Moroccan chickpeas
    with carrots
    & dates 104
chocolate
  chocolate espresso
    pots 110
  chocolate-dipped
    cherries 112
  dark chocolate 24
  cider vinegar 13
cinnamon 17
  apple, cinnamon &
    almond muesli 40
  cinnamon brioche
    with mixed
    berries 124
coconut 25
  coconut mango
    pudding 116
  tuna skewers with
    coconut & mango
    salad 90
constant hunger 29
crab
  lettuce wrappers
    with crab 82
cranberry & apple
  smoothie 64
cravings 7, 26
crêpes, light 41
cucumber
  chicken brochettes
    with cucumber
    & kelp salad 94

Dates 23
  date & banana
    pancakes 42
  Moroccan chickpeas
    with carrots
    & dates 104
digestion 7
poor 29

Eggs 18
  huevos rancheros 50
  Moroccan baked
    eggs 52
  poached eggs
    & spinach 48
  smoked haddock with
    poached eggs 92
exercise 9

Fat around the
  middle 26
fish, baked, with lemon
  grass & green
  papaya salad 93

Gazpacho, chilled 74
grapefruit 20
  ginger-grilled
    grapefruit with
    honey yogurt 44
  pumpkin curry with
    pink grapefruit
    salad 107
green tea 13
  green tea & ginger
    granita 120

High blood
  pressure 27
hormones 6
  hormone
    imbalance 29
huevos rancheros 50

Insulin 6
iodine 8

Lamb & apricot
  tagine with pearl
  barley 100
lentils 19
  butternut squash,
    rosemary and lentil
    soup 77
  lettuce wrappers
    with crab 82
liver (human body) 8
low mood 28
low self-esteem 29

Mangoes
  coconut mango
    pudding 116
  tuna skewers with
    coconut & mango
    salad 90
  menopausal weight
    gain 26
Moroccan baked
  eggs 52
Moroccan chickpeas
  with carrots
  & dates 104

Oats
  apple, cinnamon
    & almond muesli 40
  baked apples 118
  green tea porridge
    with blueberries 36
  summer berry
    granola 38
  oranges, sliced, with
    almonds 121

Pancakes, date
  & banana 42
papaya
  baked fish with lemon
    grass & green
    papaya salad 93
  raspberry, pineapple &
    papaya smoothie 65
parsnips 14
  scallop, parsnip
    & carrot salad 84
  split pea & parsnip
    soup 72
pasta, chicken &
  blueberry pasta
    salad 96
peaches
  fruity summer
    milkshake 47
  griddled peaches
    & apricots with
    honey yogurt 122
peppers, red, & feta
  rolls with olives 88
pineapple, raspberry, &
  papaya smoothie 65
pork, cheesy, with
  parsnip puree 102
post-pregnancy
  weight 26
processed foods 8

pumpkin
  pumpkin curry
    with pink grapefruit
    salad 107
  pumpkin, feta
    & pine nut salad 86
  pumpkin soup 73
  pumpkin seeds 15
  turmeric-roasted
    pumpkin seeds 54

Raspberries
  raspberry, pineapple &
    papaya smoothie 65
rice
  sushi rice salad 80
rosemary
  butternut squash,
    rosemary and lentil
    soup 77
rye 15
  Swedish rye
    cookies 66

Salmon
  asparagus with
    smoked salmon 53
  sushi rice salad 80
scallops
  scallop & broccoli
    broth 68
  scallop, parsnip
    & carrot salad 84
seaweeds 20
  chicken brochettes
    with cucumber &
    kelp salad 94
  roasted seaweed &
    sesame snack 57
sesame seeds
  baked tofu sticks 58
  chicken brochettes
    with cucumber &
    kelp salad 94
  sushi rice salad 80
sleep 8
slow metabolism 28
smoked haddock with
  poached eggs 92
smoked salmon,
  asparagus with 53
soup 7
soya 14
spinach, poached
  eggs &, 48
split pea & parsnip
  soup 72

stress 27
Swedish rye cookies 66

Thai red vegetable
  curry 108
thyroid, underactive 28
tofu
  baked tofu sticks 58
  vegetable & tofu
    stir-fry 106
tomatoes
  chilled gazpacho 74
  huevos rancheros 50
tortillas
  aubergine dip with
    toasted torillas 62
treats 8
tuna 22
  tuna pâté 61
  tuna skewers with
    coconut & mango
    salad 90
turmeric 22
  turmeric-roasted
    pumpkin seeds 54
two-week
  programme 9, 30

Vegetables
  Thai red
    vegetable curry 108
  vegetable & tofu
    stir fry 106

Weight loss 9

Yogurt
  almond & apple
    ca ke with vanilla
    yogurt 113
  blueberry cheesecake
    pots 114
  chocolate espresso
    pots 110
  ginger-grilled
    grapefruit with
    honey yogurt 44
  griddled peaches
    & apricots with
    honey yogurt 122

Acknowledgements

Gill Paul would like to
thank the very talented
team at Octopus: Denise
Bates, who came up
with the idea for the
series; Katy Denny, Alex
Stetter and Jo Wilson
who edited the books so
efficiently and made it
all work; and to the
design team of Jonathan
Christie and Isabel de
Cordova for making it all
look so gorgeous. Thank
you also to Karel Bata
for all the support and
for eating my cooking.

Karen Sullivan would
like to thank Cole, Luke
and Marcus.

Picture credits

Commissioned
photography ©
Octopus Publishing
Group/Will Heap apart
from the following:
Getty Images: Glow
Images 21; Sally Williams
Photography 9.
Octopus Publishing
Group: Stephen Conroy
69, 79; Will Heap 111, 123,
125; Lis Parsons 81, 87,
99, 101; William Shaw 49,
83, 89; Craig Robertson
75; Ian Wallace 39, 63.
Thinkstock: iStockphoto
10, 12, 14, 19, 24, 27, 28,
34; Wavebreak Media 5.